613.71   Waitz, Grete,
W   1953-

          On the run.

$19.95

DATE			

On the Run

On the Run

Exercise and Fitness for Busy People

By Grete Waitz
with Gloria Averbuch

Rodale Press, Inc.
Emmaus, Pennsylvania

Notice

This book is intended as a reference volume only, not as a medical manual. The information given here is designed to help you make informed decisions about your exercise and fitness program. It is not intended as a substitute for any professional medical or fitness advice. You should seek your doctor's approval before you begin any exercise program.

Printed in the United States of America on acid-free ∞ , recycled paper ♻

Cover and Interior Designer: Christopher R. Neyen

Cover and Interior Photographer: Mitch Mandel

Library of Congress Cataloging-in-Publication Data
Waitz, Grete, 1953–
    On the run : exercise and fitness for busy people / by Grete Waitz
with Gloria Averbuch.
        p.   cm.
    Includes index.
    ISBN 0–87596–456–7 hardcover
    1. Physical fitness. 2. Exercise. 3. Running. 4. Jogging.
I. Averbuch, Gloria, 1951–   . II. Title.
GV481.W14   1997
613.7'1—dc21   97–26320

Distributed in the book trade by St. Martin's Press

2   4   6   8   10   9   7   5   3   1   hardcover

──── OUR PURPOSE ────

*"We inspire and enable people to improve
their lives and the world around them."*

To my family, who has always loved me for who I am,
not for what I have achieved through running.
— G. W.

To Paul Friedman, world-class husband,
father, and runner.
— G. A.

Contents

Preface

In my kitchen cabinet at home in Oslo, I have a shelf where I keep matches, candles, batteries, and other assorted necessities, some of which I rarely use. Sitting with them are my medals, including those from the Olympics and the World Championships.

People are usually shocked when they hear where I keep my medals, but those who know me well only laugh. They understand how I view those prizes. Although I am enormously proud of the accomplishments they represent, I understand that they are only symbols. For me, they are like the matches and candles: items to be kept on a shelf. I know I earned those medals; I know I have them. That's enough.

To my way of thinking, past achievements are not important in and of themselves. It's what we do with those achievements that counts. I had an incredible athletic career that has spanned most of my adult life. I was fortunate to have that career, but I worked long and hard to enjoy it. And when it was over, I learned that what endured was my ability and my desire to take both the luck and the experience of hard work and create a new career in which I could do something for other people. This realization did not come easily. For a long while, I found it difficult to let go of the life I had lived for so many years. But now I am grateful that I found another, equally fulfilling mission.

My second career started at the finish line of my last race, and it revolves around my passion to educate people about the benefits of health and fitness. In a sense, I have come full circle, as I am now doing what I did before running became my sole occupation: teaching. When I speak at clinics or races, or when I write articles or create training programs, I feel the same excitement and satisfaction I felt so many years ago when a light bulb would go on over the head of one of my teenage students in Norway.

I worked hard on this book, and I am gratified by the results. As the book progressed, I began to realize that I have learned important lessons and acquired valuable information both during and since my competitive days. I know a lot of world-class athletes, and I even coach one. We are a small community of people who share our knowledge with one another. But I also want to share that knowledge with the average person.

I am confident that this is a book for everyone. If it informs and enlightens you, I will be just as proud and happy as I was when I wore each of those medals around my neck.

— Grete Waitz

Acknowledgments

Special thanks to our editor, John Reeser, who understands the power of a kind word; Gerard Hartmann, our other set of eyes; and Jack, for being Jack. I would also like to thank the numerous people who have supported my efforts, particularly my longtime sponsors adidas and Chase Manhattan Bank, who have enabled me to spread the word about running and fitness.

Introduction

Initially, Grete Waitz didn't want to write another book. She and I had already written one together—*World Class*, in 1984. It isn't that she shuns work. Far from it. Grete is one of the hardest workers I know—as an athlete, a scholar, and an author. In fact, if you want to understand what made her a great runner, look back to her school days in Norway, where she graduated first in her class and was the youngest student to be admitted to a very competitive teachers college.

Grete told me that she didn't want to write another book because she thought she had nothing new to offer. The subject seemed so obvious to her. I could only smile. That's because I knew that the woman who rewrote the record books, almost single-handedly defined women's road running, and is one of the world's most respected champions also is a great teacher and powerful advocate for health and fitness.

Everyone reveres Grete Waitz. But it is not just her accomplishments that move me. It is the quality and class that define her work and her life. It is the personal choices she makes—the countless people and projects to which she selflessly devotes her time and energy. It is her sense of humor, wisdom, grace, and humility. Good authors are people who have something valuable to share, and Grete has so much.

No one has used her running and sports experience more meaningfully than Grete Waitz. This was most dramatically evident in her 1992 New York City Marathon run with her friend and mentor, the late Fred Lebow. With Grete serving as his coach, Fred trained for and completed the marathon while in remission from brain cancer. Grete not only designed a training program for Fred but also ran his race with him every step of the way. Both of them shed tears of emotion during the final miles.

Running behind the two, I could see the effort it took Grete to go at

Fred's pace. Ironically, the slow cadence caused her severe muscle soreness for days afterward. But mostly what I saw was Grete Waitz at her finest.

I will always remember the display of love and generosity she showed our mutual friend Fred. It is a measure of the woman, and the athlete.

When I talk about knowing and working with Grete, I always find myself using one phrase: She elevates me. I am a better person for knowing her, sharing her life, recording her words. It isn't a job to write a book with her; it is a gift. And I knew, as she worked so diligently to express the depth of her knowledge about and passion for exercise and fitness, that she was, in her usual fashion, giving a great gift to the readers of this book.

— Gloria Averbuch

Advice to Get You Going

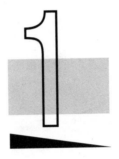

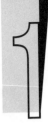

The Life and Times of Grete Waitz
Insights from a Champion

I was 12 years old when I first joined a local sports club in Oslo. I had absolutely no plans to be a world-class athlete. I was just one of the millions of Norwegians who join these clubs and participate in a variety of activities, from track and field to soccer, skiing, and hiking.

For the next few years, I took part in some competitions—shot put, long jump, sprints—but I didn't win anything. That didn't stop me from participating. It was so much fun, and the atmosphere was great. The local sports club was the social focus of all the young people. Soon after I joined, I was introduced to one of the older boys, who later became one of my running mates. His name was Jack Waitz, and he eventually became my husband.

Actually, my first runs were behind my house. I wore an old pair of spikes I found lying around. (They must have been from World War II!) When I decided to get more serious, I had to find a sports club, since the schools had no programs. My older brother Jan, who belonged to a track-and-field club for boys only, helped me to find one

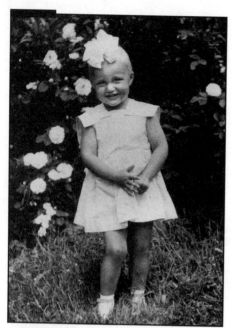

I was groomed to be the "perfect little girl," but it didn't last!

that accepted girls. Little did I realize, as a girlfriend and I walked to the club that first day, how much the Vidar Sports Club would change my life. Here is where I discovered and developed both my athletic talent and my love of physical activity. Years later, I am still an active member of Vidar.

At age 14, I placed third in a 500-meter cross-country race. It was the first time I had run more than a 100-meter dash. That was the start of my career. Soon after, my brother Arild built my first trophy case. At age 16, I became the Norwegian National Junior Champion in the 400 meters and 800 meters. Soon after that, I got the thrill of my life when I took my first trip outside Scandinavia for a competition.

When I look back on my youth, I see it as an ideal basis for my athletic career. Norwegians place a high value on nature and outdoor sports, and the 10,000 sports clubs, to which more than one-third of the population belongs, are part of a common atmosphere that also reinforces a healthy lifestyle. These clubs are a way of life in Norway and many other European countries. They specialize in many different sports and function as community centers for children and their parents.

Most Norwegians are physically active on a regular basis. I didn't consider what I did at the club "training." Being physically active was a pleasure, and doing a variety of activities early on gave me a versatile and physically fit body. This active lifestyle was the first brick I put down for the foundation of my career.

Today things are different. Even in Norway, because of the distractions of modern life, it is difficult to get young people involved in sports. In the United States, the situation is far worse. From what I have observed, a small percentage of young people in the United States get channeled early on into one sport. This approach may limit their physical development and increase their chances of burning out or dropping out because of participation limits. The rest of America's youths generally fall victim to a more sedentary lifestyle. Looking back, I guess I was lucky. We didn't have a television in my house until I was 10. I had no choice but to play outside and be active.

Although Norwegians prize fitness and sports, becoming a female athlete, not to mention a professional one, was not easy. We, too, have our social prejudices and stereotypes. In my childhood, piano lessons were my dreaded fate. After two sons, my parents finally had a daughter—who they hoped would live up to their image of a girl. They insisted that I take piano lessons and wear pink dresses with matching ribbons tied in my carefully curled blond hair. Ultimately, this was not to be. The ribbons fell out, and the dresses got dirty when I played outside. My mother told me to behave like a girl. That meant sitting quietly and playing with dolls. But I was always running and playing with the boys.

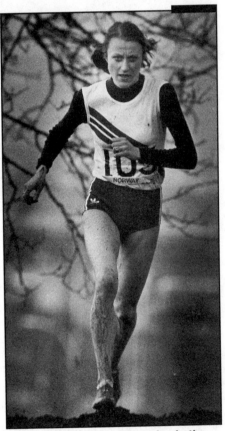

On my way to one of five wins in the World Cross-Country Championships. This was my first, in 1978 in Glasgow, Scotland.

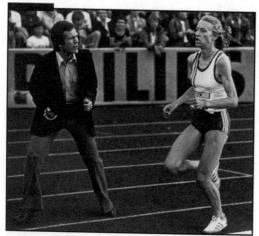

Seeing my husband, Jack, and the look on my face, you can appreciate what it takes to break a world record. On July 17, 1979, I did just that—running the 3000 meters in 8:31.7.

Maybe that's why I continued to do so as an adult.

I was a good student and a fairly obedient child, but I also was very active. I was intent on developing my running. After I won several running awards, my mother made a comment (which she doesn't remember) that served to fuel my athletic aspirations even more. "Why bother with all this running?" she asked. "You're not going to be a running star anyway." It was a bitter moment for me, and I stormed out of the house. When I became the Norwegian Junior Champion, my parents realized that I was serious. They even bought me some sports gear, and, more important, they let me stop taking piano lessons!

For my entire career, athletics and a healthy lifestyle went hand in hand. I took that healthy lifestyle for granted. It wasn't until I came to the United States for the first time that I realized a healthy lifestyle isn't the norm. It first hit me when I ordered what I thought was a Scandinavian breakfast—typically whole-grain bread with perhaps some cheese and jam. When my order of "Danish" came, I looked down in shock at a basket of sugary pastry.

Fairly early in my career, I became interested in the mental-physical connection inherent in my running. I was attending teachers college in Norway and was often very tired from studying. I noticed how my fatigue, stress, and grumpiness would disappear after I trained. It was as if I were a new person, filled with energy.

In the 1970s, I learned the hard way how to strike a balance between a job and a sports career. For nearly half my career, through two

Olympic Games, I was a middle school teacher as well as a competitor. While training for the 1976 Olympics, I had to juggle twice-a-day running around 2 hours of daily commuting and my teaching job. It wasn't until 1980 that I quit my job and started running full-time.

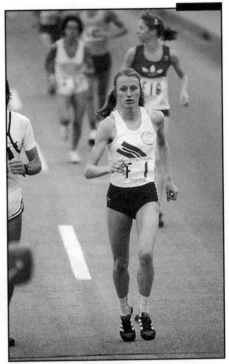

After I began running the marathon, I realized how strong the lifestyle-sports connection is. In 1978, on the night before my first marathon, I had a meal that broke all the prerace rules. I knew nothing about "carbo loading" or taking in enough fluids. We were in New York, celebrating. I am embarrassed to say that I broke a world record the day after a dinner of shrimp

In my second marathon, New York City in 1979, I became the first woman ever to break 2:30.

cocktail, filet mignon, a glass of wine, and ice cream. Two years later, at a New York City restaurant, I noticed another marathoner eating a plate of spaghetti. He recognized me and came over. Looking at my plate, he asked, somewhat surprised, "You're going to run a marathon?" Apparently, I wasn't eating the "right" thing.

My running roots were planted in the track, then branched out to the roads. Although tennis and other sports enjoyed a wave of popularity, road running—accessible to nearly everyone—was where the fitness boom truly began. The marathon fever of the early 1980s got a lot of people into running and a lot of others more physically active. When the road running boom peaked and then leveled off, in came walking and then cross-training. Now a second running boom is sweeping America. Whereas the first boom consisted of runners trying to break 3

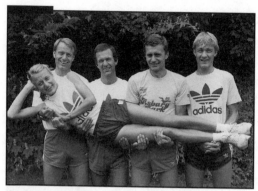

My "support crew," from left to right: brother Jan; husband, Jack; brother Arild; and nephew Geir.

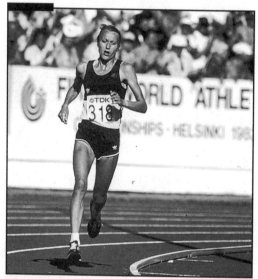

The World Championship Marathon in Helsinki, Finland in 1983. My "dream race"—the day everything came together, and I felt invincible.

hours in the marathon, the second seems to be driven mostly by middle-age people who want to reap the health benefits of running.

Today I include cross-training as part of my exercise program. I still run, but several times a week I bike, walk, work out on a cross-country ski machine, or use a pool for deep-water running. I meet many "retired" runners who still work out. They may not do marathons, but they want to keep the good feeling that comes from exercise.

When you are a world-class runner, you want to be the best. You must follow a very narrow, intense path to reach your goal. To be the best runner, you must run a lot and run hard. You can't even allow yourself to cross-train unless you get injured and have no choice. An athlete doesn't run more than 100 miles a week to be healthy; she does it because she wants to be the best runner in the world.

When I was racing, I pushed myself as hard as I could without going over the edge. The key was to train as much as my body could absorb without breaking down. Now I feel healthier because I don't train as much or as hard. With my current training, overuse injuries are a thing of the past. I also can take a rest when I feel like it without worrying about losing my edge over other elite runners.

I had a wonderful athletic career that spanned more than two decades. I still treasure every minute

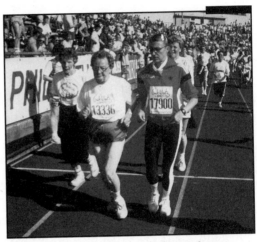

It was a big moment in our lives when my Mom and I finished the Grete Waitz Run.

of it. But when I retired from competition in 1990, I realized that there was no reason for me to run every day. I'm no longer concerned with being the best in the world. Now I am more concerned with being a healthy, strong, and productive person. I want to live a quality life and continue to run, hike, and bike into my fifties, sixties, and beyond.

After my retirement from competition, I began to work more regularly in the area of health and fitness. Since 1986, I have been a spokesperson for the Chase Corporate Challenge. In that role, I travel around the United States and Europe meeting thousands of busy working people who are concerned about fitness. As a representative for adidas, Polar (maker of heart rate monitors), and NordicTrack at fitness clinics and race expos, I meet many more of these people.

I also am very involved in organizing my own race. Before a statue of me was unveiled in front of Oslo's Bislett Stadium, I was asked how the event should be commemorated. Inspired by my experiences as a young girl who loved sports and as a woman runner, I started the Grete Waitz Run for women. It began in 1984 with a surprising turnout of 3,000. Today, to my astonishment and satisfaction, the annual 5-K run draws 45,000 women—this in a country of only four million!

A Unique Perspective

Over the years, I have observed how different American society is from my own. Because I now divide my time between the United States and Norway, I see the contrast of the two cultures most acutely.

I applaud the intentions of people in the United States. They truly seem to want to become fit. They read, study, and experiment with their exercise, and they are very public about motivating others to get fit. But as an outsider looking in, I also recognize the difficulties that Americans face.

Unfortunately, Americans live in a society of contradictions. On the one hand, there is a great deal of discussion about the need for physical exercise. Americans need and want to lose weight and get into shape. On the other hand, this country does everything possible to limit physical activity—all in the name of convenience. In most countries, you walk to the bank, do housework, and garden. In the United States, you drive up to the bank window, hire a housekeeper, and cut your grass with a power mower. If you walk, people think something is wrong. Often during my walks in the United States, drivers stop and ask me if I need a ride. Some cities don't even have any sidewalks.

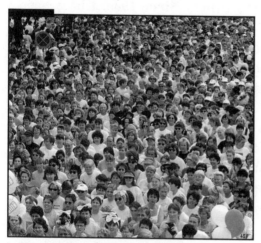

I still get chills watching 45,000 women take off in the Grete Waitz Run.

Another problem is that Americans are constantly pitched the quick fix. Advertising promises fast and easy everything, including fitness. People are taught that getting into shape and losing weight are instantaneous. Almost every television commercial and advertisement makes it look that way. I find this appalling. In Norway, before any such advertisement can be aired or published, such claims must be proved.

Because of this quick fix trend in American society, I understand how difficult it is to see health and fitness as a natural part of life and an area that requires work. When I speak about fitness, I tell Americans that they have to be aware of these problems, and I try to support their efforts to change their attitudes and habits in

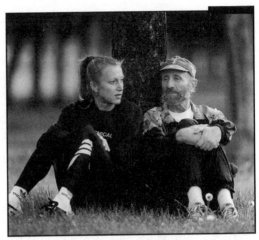

My friend and mentor, Fred Lebow, the late New York City Marathon director.

such a hostile environment. People get set in their ways. I understand that it is probably just as hard for most people to imagine training at the crack of dawn as it is for me to imagine not doing so.

The United States also is a country of extremes. Sometimes it seems that people are either totally sedentary, existing solely on fast food, or totally committed to a health regimen, eating plain pasta and sports bars and running marathons. It's hard for many people to take the middle road. I want to show Americans how they can live fit and healthy lives without taking the term "endurance exercise" too literally. I want them to know that they don't have to be as thin as a world-class marathoner or as muscular as a sprinter. They can lead normal lives, even carry a few extra pounds, and still be fit and healthy—even athletic.

From my lifelong participation in sports and fitness, I know all the angles. I have talked with and worked with many people who have faced every imaginable challenge and have overcome great obstacles. When I think of busy people fitting in exercise, my Norwegian friend Ketil Moe comes to mind. Ketil, who is in his late twenties and suffers from cystic fibrosis, needs several hours just to walk or run a few miles. He must physically prepare himself (by clearing his lungs) for at least an hour before leaving the house, and he requires a long postexercise rest when he gets home. But he still trained for and completed the New York City Marathon 10 times. I have always felt that if Ketil—who is an inspiration to me and all of Norway—can do it, the rest of us surely can.

I have met many incredible people who have given me the inspiration to work for health and fitness and have helped me to understand that exercise is our best celebration of life. Like all of us, my feelings have been formed by many experiences. At age 18, I was in love with one of my older Vidar club mates, who was my training partner and coach. When he became ill and went to the hospital, I just assumed that he would get well and we would live happily ever after. But in the month I sat at his hospital bedside, doing my homework as he slept, I watched his formerly athletic body waste away. He was dying from cancer.

I was inconsolable for months after my boyfriend died. I grew thin from not eating, and then ill. A group of friends from the Vidar Sports

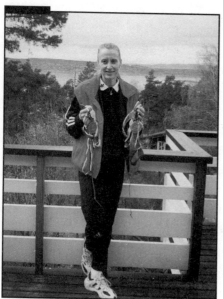

My medals make a rare trip out of my kitchen cabinet.

Club slowly brought me back to myself by taking me back to the club. I used running to help me move on. I know that sports and fitness can help people get through hard times. Exercise is one constant that can take you away from your problems, big or small, even if only temporarily.

In 1992, many years after my friend died, I ran along the streets of New York City with Fred Lebow, my friend and the man behind the New York City Marathon. Fred was in remission from brain cancer and was running his own five-borough race for the first time. It was his way of affirming life and good health. We ran the 26 miles together, with me serving as his coach. The emotion of the race was so strong that we both cried as we ran the last few miles. I never got my tenth victory at New York, but that day with Fred was a victory in itself. Although he died in 1994, I feel that his spirit is with me. It is especially strong when I run in Central Park. Now I am proud to be the coach of Fred's Team, an all-comers group that runs all over the world to raise money for cancer research at Memorial Sloan-Kettering Cancer Center in New York City, which is where Fred received treatment.

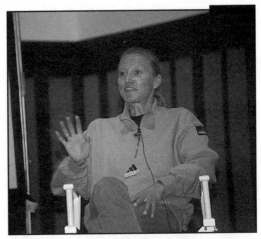

I enjoy my "new career" as a clinic speaker and health and fitness educator. Actually, it's like returning to my old career as a teacher.

Even the most casual exercisers have incidents that move and inspire them. I know the feeling of joy from conquering the challenges, the ups and downs of getting fit, and the struggle to maintain that fitness. And I know that being fit and healthy does contribute to being a happy, fulfilled person, despite the fact that, at times, the endeavor can seem challenging or difficult. This book will educate you not only on how to become fit but also on how to enjoy exercise and integrate it into your daily life. If you are already an exerciser, it will help you to become a better, stronger, and more educated one.

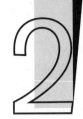

Motivation and Goals
A Pep Talk from Coach Grete

Very often in the running clinics I conduct, people ask, "How do I get motivated? How do I get inspired? How do I get disciplined?" They follow up their questions by telling me how difficult these qualities are to acquire. I'll say it right up front: There is no magic recipe. Too many people I meet believe that you can sit in a chair and be given motivation. With exercise and fitness, you get it by doing.

The mental qualities you need are all linked like a chain. If you give exercise a try and see results, even if it's as simple as feeling good that you got out the door, you'll become motivated to repeat the experience. Seeing results is inspiring. As for discipline, the more often you do the activity, the more you become disciplined. Eventually, exercise will become a habit, like brushing your teeth, and you won't need as much discipline to work out.

If you have been sedentary, getting into shape and losing weight will not be easy. Doing so will mean changing your habits, and I know how hard it is to change habits. I still have habits from my competitive running days that I can't break. I get up at the crack of dawn, even though I don't have to, despite my occasional attempts to sleep in.

After I retired, it was very difficult for me to get out of the training rhythm I'd been following all my adult life. I had to change gradually. For the first year, I still ran twice a day a couple of times a week. By the second year, I cut back to seven to nine weekly sessions. Only by the third year did I manage to adjust to training just once a day. People still approach me when I'm on the bike at my health club and ask me why I'm biking so hard. Working out hard is a habit of mine.

For your exercise and fitness to become lifelong, your motivation must come from within. If you exercise to please your spouse or your friends, or if you have unrealistic expectations, your change of habits and resolve will not last. Even those blessed with talent must get their motivation from within. In my coaching over the years, I have worked with some topflight runners who were motivated for the wrong reason. They ran to please their parents or their coach. At best, this is a short-term motivator.

If you don't enjoy what you do, it probably won't last. When I first began running, I wasn't a success. I usually finished in the back third of the pack, and my parents didn't really encourage me. But I truly enjoyed running, so I kept at it. In time, success motivated me to work at excelling. The point is that although your motivation may change, you still must be self-motivated.

Remember that most things that are satisfying and enjoyable come from working hard. Once you begin the training outlined in this book, you will have taken the first steps toward gaining the mental edge to make your fitness a lifelong habit. When you get used to being fit, you'll want to keep that feeling. That, in itself, is a tremendous motivation.

Here are some tips on motivation that I've found successful over the years.

Make the decision to exercise and set a goal. Whether it means basic fitness or running a race, decide what you want to do. Clearly define that goal and use it as a guiding light to keep you moving forward. Even as a teenager, I was determined to develop my running.

Set aside the time. Too many irregular exercisers work out on impulse. They do it when they feel like it or when they can find the time.

Exercise is most likely to happen if it is a definite appointment you keep with yourself. My appointment is every morning half an hour after I wake up, and I try never to miss it.

Make exercise a priority. You'll keep your appointment if you have decided it is important. In my competitive days, I never allowed anything or anyone to interfere with my running. Even today, I find a way to structure my appointments and obligations around my exercise.

Add value to your workouts. If you exercise with your children, family, or friends, your relationships will become stronger. When I began to walk and jog with my mother, she was 65 years old. We had some of our most meaningful talks while exercising. I know those conversations wouldn't have occurred while we were sitting at the kitchen table.

Form a group. Some of the 45,000 women who participate in the Grete Waitz Run in Norway are matched up to train together. By training with friends or people at the same fitness level, you're more likely to stay with your exercise program. You end up motivating each other. On days when one member of the group doesn't feel like working out, other members are there to give a little push.

Goals

I don't stress goals; I stress health. But I do realize that goals can be an effective motivator. Some people don't need concrete goals. More abstract goals, such as achieving good health, are motivation enough. Other people are motivated more by specific goals. If you are sedentary, for example, setting a definite goal, such as losing 15 pounds in six months, might be your key to making it happen. If you reach your goal, you can reward yourself by buying new clothes. If you decide to set goals, be sure to keep several important things in mind.

Flexibility. Although many fitness experts stress having goals, many things can happen to interfere with them. Life is unpredictable. The danger with goals is that you may end up feeling like a failure if you don't reach them. If you do set goals, you have to be flexible. It's okay to adjust them. If you allow yourself flexibility, when something

The Good and the Bad

Good goals—those with a better than average chance of being realized—are specific, reasonable, and achievable within a definite time frame. For example: "In two months, I want to lose 10 pounds and be in shape to walk a local 5-K race. To do so, I'm going to follow the beginning exercise program and adopt the eating tips in this book." Mentally prepare by visualizing yourself crossing the finish line during that 5-K.

Bad goals involve going at full speed, but in the wrong direction. "I want to look like I did in high school" is not a bad goal in and of itself, but you're unlikely to reach it because it is vague. You could be in this situation, with an unfulfilled goal, for years.

A bad goal also can be unrealistic. Say your best time in a marathon is 3:30, and your goal is to run 3 hours (a significant improvement). If you run 3:15, that represents positive, significant progress. But according to your goal, you are a failure.

Set goals that you can achieve. Having goals is positive; they become negative only when they are too ambitious to be reached.

occurs that causes you to postpone a goal, you won't be tempted to fall off the wagon altogether.

Balance. One of the runners I coach on Fred's Team (a group that runs the New York City Marathon) has a full-time job and a new baby, yet he is as serious as a professional about his training and running goals. His wife once commented that she didn't know how long she could endure the strain this was creating in their lives. I also am pretty sure that he is not as productive in his job as he could be.

I had a similar experience early in my career when my goal was very ambitious for the life I was leading. I trained longer and harder than I ever had for the 1500 meters at the 1976 Olympics. I was up against the Soviet women, and I would have to fly to beat them. My goal was to make the finals.

A photo of my heat shows five women abreast at the tape, all finishing within two-tenths of a second of each other. I ran a personal best (4:04) and set a Scandinavian record, but I still placed only seventh. I failed to make the finals and was given a hard time by the Norwegian newspapers, even though my heat was later protested because it included too many of the favorites.

Although I knew it had been quite an accomplishment to get as far as I had (that photo made *The Guinness Book of Records*), I was bitterly disappointed. In retrospect, however, I am proud of what I managed to do. I realize now that I had loaded stress on top of stress. In addition to the training, I was commuting a long way to my job and working hard as a new teacher, determined to make a name for myself. From 1974 to 1976, I didn't miss one day of training. Some weeks, I logged up to 125 miles, and there were many days when I would cry from fatigue.

It's important to draw a distinct line between being a recreational exerciser and being a professional, or even a serious, athlete. During my running career, my life consisted of eating, sleeping, and running. But even a committed professional has to accept the fact that sometimes other aspects of life intervene. Once, during a several-month span, I took care of my nephews while my sister-in-law was hospitalized with a serious illness. The stress was too great, and I experienced a breakdown in my training.

Tolerance. Don't make goals synonymous with guilt. Through my work with the Chase Corporate Challenge, I meet many runners who complain about how difficult it is to stay with their fitness routines. They express the guilt they feel if they skip a workout. If you miss exercising now and then, you're not a failure. Too many people put this pressure on themselves. Their expectations are unreasonable. They don't understand that a moderate amount of exercise is all they need to stay healthy. They're too "big-goal" oriented.

Reasonable expectations. I am all for taking on the challenge of serious running or racing. But I am wary of people who focus too strongly on a specific time or a particularly high risk event like the marathon. The chances of something going wrong are so much greater than for an athlete who is obsessed about a sport. That's why I'm not crazy about the idea of magazines publishing the running schedules of elite athletes. It creates a false impression of what training should be for the average person. Those articles should come with a warning: Undertake any part of this training program at your own risk!

Many people have the wrong idea about what constitutes an average amount of exercise. I often talk to runners who say, "I don't run very much." When I inquire about what not very much is, they often answer, "Five miles." For the majority of people, 5 miles is quite a long way. You have to be pretty fit and dedicated to run that far. When I tell people that 30 to 40 minutes of running several times a week is enough to keep them fit, they seem surprised at the small amount. Yet, it can be that easy.

When you map out that 5-mile course, ask yourself what your goal is. Don't pay any attention to that old adage: "No pain, no gain." Exercise doesn't have to be painful, long, or disruptive of your life to be beneficial. First and foremost, your exercise goal should be enjoyment and good health.

An example of positive goal setting comes from my career as a marathoner. Miracles don't happen in the marathon; it's a very "realistic" event. What you do in a marathon is a direct result of the work you put in. After I set a world record in my first marathon, there was a lot of publicity about how the longest I had ever run in training before the event was a mere 12 miles. People failed to realize that I had come into that event as a world-class track runner, not a novice jogger. That means that although I had run no longer than 12 miles at any one time, I had been doing overall high-mileage and high-intensity training.

Being realistic was one of my strengths in the marathon. I always set my goals according to my training and latest race results. I approached important races with a strategy in mind. Sometimes the results were better than my expectations. Sometimes, because of weather, for instance, I was forced to change my goals. Because I was prepared and willing to be flexible, the outcome of my races made sense.

The marathon also is instructive because of its difficulty. It has to be a goal you truly want to achieve. Having goals is important, but they are useful only if you believe in them wholeheartedly and identify yourself with them. You should set your goals yourself and for yourself. Your fitness, weight loss, or competitive goals should not belong to a coach or a spouse. They should be your creation, and when you succeed, they will be your achievement.

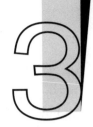

Body Basics
Knowing What Makes You Tick

Being knowledgeable about how to achieve a goal goes a long way toward motivating you to reach it. I also believe that if you have a basic understanding of how your body functions when you exercise, you will go a lot further with your fitness program. Just by answering questions such as how hard and how long to exercise and what happens to your body when you work out will help you set good goals. Whatever your goal or fitness level, you'll know better how to home in on it.

Even serious athletes may have a motivational or training problem that can be solved by understanding how their bodies work. They may reach a plateau in their training and feel that they aren't getting enough back from what they are putting in. Perhaps someone's running times don't improve, or the person has trouble keeping off weight. Proper heart rate monitoring during training and balanced muscle strength and flexibility can help athletes improve their training and, if necessary, rededicate themselves to the sport.

I am not an expert in physiology, although I have worked with many people who are. I do know what concerns the average person regarding fitness, the body, and exercise, however. I've chosen the following topics and information based on the discussions I have had over the years with athletes and exercisers on every level and from all walks of life.

The Heart of the Matter

The heart is the most important muscle in the body. It powers the lungs and the circulatory system, and it is the key to health and fitness. The heart also is the best gauge of the effectiveness of exercise. Specifically, your heart rate helps to determine the proper amount and intensity of exercise.

In the past few years, some experts have advocated judging the level of exercise intensity by perceived exertion, or how your body feels. They believe that this is both simpler than measuring heart rate and sufficiently effective. I am all for keeping exercise simple, but I do think that perceived exertion is too subjective a measure and that people often do not have the correct perception regarding their exercise. Whether you are a beginner or an advanced exerciser, what you perceive as hard may be in your mind, not your body. Likewise, you may think you are taking it easy, but in reality your body isn't.

For most of my career, I never measured my heart rate. When heart rate monitors first became popular, I didn't think I needed one. After all, my experienced perception was my monitor. When I finally tried one and got an accurate measure of my heart rate, I learned a lot. For one thing, I was running too fast on my easy days. For another, my rest between periods of intense effort on my hard runs was too short. I needed to slow my pace so that the essential recovery process could occur. The more I learned about heart rate, the more I realized how effective a gauge it is. Using it, I was able to train more correctly, without the guesswork involved in my own perceptions. Monitoring my heart rate also helped me not to overtrain, which I had a habit of doing. Now I require all the athletes I coach to wear a heart rate monitor. It allows me to custom-design the proper training program for each one of them.

I highly recommend that all exercisers measure their heart rate as a way to make training safe and efficient. You can do it manually or with a heart rate monitor. A heart rate monitor is easy to use and accurate. It also can be a great motivator. As you become fitter, you'll see tangible and precise results. Your heart rate will go down, and your recovery after exertion will improve, since your strengthened heart will not have to work as hard.

You also can take your pulse manually. When I don't use a monitor, I often stop to calculate my heart rate manually just as a check. To do this, use the two fingers next to the thumb (not the thumb, which has less sensitivity because of its thick skin) and place them on either side of your throat or on the inside of either wrist below the thumb line. Move your fingers slightly until you feel the strongest beat. I find that the most accurate measure is to count for 6 seconds and multiply by 10 to get the number of beats per minute. The resting heart rate range for an inactive person is about 68 to 78 beats per minute (bpm); for a fit person, it's below 62 bpm.

Fitness Facts

A sedentary person's heart beats
- 75 times per minute
- 4,500 times per hour
- 108,000 times per day

A regular exerciser's heart beats
- 55 times per minute
- 3,300 times per hour
- 79,200 times per day

In a year, an inactive person's heart beats 10,512,000 times more than an active person's heart!

Who doesn't relate to the importance—the strength as well as the fragility—of the human heart? That's why I like to flash these facts up on a big screen when I do my fitness clinics. Look at all the extra work an unfit heart has to do. It's pretty scary but also very effective. I may cause people to feel guilty, but at least I make them aware of why they should be doing aerobic exercise.

The heart is a muscle about the size of your fist. It can do amazing things, but if you don't work it, it will get weaker. If you do work it, it will get stronger. But it won't stay that way if you don't keep it in shape. One of the most common comments I hear from people everywhere is, "I used to work out." Exercise is not like money you put in the bank and withdraw when you need it. It doesn't gain interest either. To reap its benefits, exercise must become, and remain, a regular part of your lifestyle.

Whether you measure your heart rate manually or use a monitor, you must determine your maximum heart rate (MHR) before you can figure out your ideal heart rate range during exercise. MHR is the rate at which your heart can't pump any harder. If you are over age 35 and out of shape, you should consult a doctor before undertaking any test or exercise program. Here is how to calculate your MHR.

MHR = 205 − Half your age (in years)

For example, the MHR for a 40-year-old should be about 185 beats per minute (205-20). But this is just a very general guideline. You also should be aware that MHR may vary by as many as 30 to 40 beats either way, depending on the individual, without implying any health problems.

With a doctor or health professional's approval, you can have your MHR tested on a bicycle or treadmill. This is, of course, the safest and most accurate method, but it's not necessary if you are healthy and fit.

Another, less extreme way to test your heart rate is to have a sub-maximal heart rate test. This is a less stressful test that does not require an all-out effort. The submax test is commonly administered by trainers or sports medicine experts at fitness centers. In fact, many gyms and fitness centers require you to take this test upon joining. Even without joining, you may be able to make an appointment to take the test at one of these places.

The recommended heart rate range for moderate, endurance-building exercise is 70 to 80 percent of MHR. Anything above 80 percent of MHR is anaerobic, or without oxygen. Interval training, which involves faster, more intense bursts of effort, followed by recovery, is anaerobic. The purpose of interval training is to enhance athletic performance. Average people who train for health and fitness do not need to work out in this range. They should expect to train three to five times a week at the moderate level for at least two months before improving their stamina. After that, they'll need to continue this amount of exercise at the moderate level to maintain their conditioning.

The moderate exercise range can be broken down into two other categories. Depending on your exercise goals, you can tailor your workouts appropriately.

Healthy heart zone is 60 to 70 percent of MHR. Training in this zone will strengthen your heart and help it to pump oxygen-rich blood to your muscles more efficiently.

Aerobic zone is 70 to 80 percent of MHR. This is also known as the *endurance-building zone*. Training in this zone benefits not only your heart but also your respiratory system.

Keeping Tabs on Your Heart

A heart rate monitor provides you with immediate feedback on how fast your heart is beating. It consists of two parts: a transmission belt strapped around the chest and a receiver (watch) on the wrist. The belt uses an electromagnetic field to relay the heart rate signal to the watch, which continuously displays the heart rate in beats per minute. Heart rate monitors are lightweight and waterproof. They are available at sporting goods stores for about $100.

If you monitor your heart rate frequently, you will become familiar with your own relative values. Experiment by taking your pulse in the morning before getting out of bed, at various times during the day, and while exercising. Changes in your usual heart rate signal changes in your fitness level. As you become fitter, your resting pulse will slow and your recovery time (the time it takes your heart rate to return to normal after exertion) will improve.

You also can use your heart rate as a guide to monitor recovery from your training load. For example, an elevated resting pulse taken first thing in the morning before getting out of bed may mean you are fatigued or ill. Five beats above the normal resting pulse is okay, but 10 to 15 beats higher is a sign of fatigue, possible illness, overtraining, too little sleep, or too much caffeine or alcohol.

The Importance of Recovery

It is necessary to focus on developing other muscles in addition to aerobic (heart and lung) conditioning. This is particularly crucial as we age, since there is a natural loss of muscle mass. But the great thing about exercise is that, to a degree, it can help you "beat the clock" by maintaining fitness, including muscle mass.

Muscle conditioning takes more work as we grow older, but it also takes on added importance. Experts believe that increased muscle mass helps both men and women to protect their bones as they age. When bones are not stressed, they lose density. This loss of density can lead to problems such as osteoporosis in later years. Weight-bearing activities such as running, walking, step aerobics, and jumping rope stimulate bone building. But the best type of activity for bones is resistance exercise (weight training), since it strengthens the muscles surrounding the bones in addition to stimulating bone building.

It is important to understand how a muscle is made stronger. It's not training that builds a muscle; training actually breaks it down. It is the act of muscle rebuilding—the recovery process—that makes it stronger. Put another way, stress breaks down tissue. Your body has the innate ability to adapt and get stronger, provided the stress isn't too great. This is where aerobic conditioning comes in. Powerful lungs deliver oxygen to the bloodstream more effectively, and a strong heart pumps oxygen-rich blood to oxygen-hungry muscles more efficiently.

Because recovery is so important to muscle building, it has to be a principal component of any exercise program. The need to recover is something that all exercisers, even the most serious athletes, often lose sight of. This rebuilding process also requires good lifestyle habits, such as getting enough sleep and maintaining a nutritious diet.

Fat Burners

If you are trying to lose or maintain weight, building muscle is the key. Just think of how much younger people eat while not gaining weight and how men can eat more than women without putting on the pounds. Although neither young people nor men are immune to the negative effects of a sedentary lifestyle, they typically have more muscle and, therefore, a higher metabolism. The bottom line is they burn fat faster.

The aging process involves more than just wrinkled skin and gray hair. Those are outward signs of aging. Inwardly, from the mid-thirties on, our ability to regenerate muscle diminishes, tissue becomes less elastic, and we lose muscle mass. As we age, our "calorie furnace" (the muscles) becomes less efficient. That is why younger people can get away with less exercise and more eating.

The scale is not always the best way to measure your true fitness. Even fit people, or those without a weight problem, make the mistake of believing that if they maintain their weight, they also maintain their fitness. This is not the case. You can weigh the same and still have lost muscle mass. A 25-year-old and a 55-year-old can both weigh 145 pounds, but the older person might look heavier, or less muscular. Similarly, you can maintain your weight, or even increase it, and look leaner. That is because muscle weighs more than fat. The best way to examine your progress from exercising is to look in the mirror or check your waist size.

On average, men have 17 percent body fat and women have 25 percent. Fat is important; we need it to survive. But fat also is inert baggage. It's muscle that helps burn calories. I like to think of muscle as being like Pac-Man, the video game character. The more muscle you have, the more Pac-Men you have, and the more they gobble up the calories.

How fast the Pac-Men move, or how fast you burn calories, depends on your metabolism. Metabolism, which is the process whereby you produce energy, depends on your genes and personal history. During exercise, your metabolism is higher and calories are burned faster. Dieting can slow your metabolism by tricking your body into conserving energy because of reduced food intake.

Much has been written about exercise creating an *afterburn* effect. The theory is that a revved-up metabolism resulting from exercise maintains an elevated resting metabolic rate (RMR) after exercise is finished. Studies show that the metabolic rate of increase is directly related to the intensity of the exercise. Resistance (weight) training and intense (interval) training produce higher increases for longer sustained periods of time, as compared to, say, walking or light jogging. You will have an elevated RMR with activities such as walking, but only for a few minutes to a few hours. In contrast, weight training can elevate RMR up to 15 hours after the workout. The same effect can be achieved with interval training.

I don't think the afterburn effect is very significant for most people, as they don't do the intense training described above. I think it is better to concentrate on building muscle. The possible benefits of afterburn are insignificant when compared to the effect of increased calorie burning because of increased muscle mass.

Creating balanced muscle strength also is important. Many exercisers have a tendency to focus on one type of exercise, usually because they enjoy it. This tendency results in developing only those muscles used in the exercise. For instance, most runners have a well-developed lower body and an underdeveloped upper body. The primary benefit of balanced muscle development (and muscle development in general) is injury prevention. In addition, not only will you perform better and burn more calories, but you also will look better.

Make Weight Loss a Reality

Let's face it, nearly everyone who exercises does so at least in part to lose or maintain weight. In times past, the rigors of daily life were enough to do that job, but not anymore.

"Don't think about diets." That's one of the first things I tell people at my clinics. You can't live on a diet for the rest of your life. Think about permanent changes in the way you eat and combine those changes with exercise. Diets do work when you consider their job is to help you shed a few pounds in the short term by restricting calories. But in most cases, a diet by itself will not keep the weight off.

We all need to adapt our eating habits as we age. What you can eat at age 45 is different from what you could eat at 25. When my husband, Jack, was in his twenties, he ate hot dogs, pizza, and a lot more junk food than he allows himself now that he is 50. This change is a function of both exercise and age. We aren't as hungry as we get older because our metabolism slows down after age 30, unless we maintain a significant level of exercise.

Even though I have adapted my eating habits over the years, I basically have the same diet. Of course, I don't eat as much now as when I was competing, but I still eat the same kinds of healthy foods. I am not as hungry from running 35 to 40 miles a week as I was when I ran more than 100 miles a week. When I was training hard and running to perform, I had to be careful to eat enough and also to eat at the right times of day. An athlete is like a race car. You have to fuel the body not just for the short run but also for long-term, optimal performance. When I was competing, I ate "premium fuel" to train and race, even if I wasn't particularly hungry. In that sense, I had the opposite problem of most people. I wasn't forced to restrict; I needed to add food. Now I can eat when I'm hungry and stop when I'm satisfied.

To help your body use food most efficiently and to lose or maintain weight, consider the following tips.

Choose wisely, and you can eat more. Go for low-calorie, low-fat foods instead of those with fewer rewards. Several big plates of salad or a baked potato can be far more satisfying than a muffin, for example, which has very little bulk or nutrition for its size and calories. When preparing meals or dining out, limit the sauces and other fat-laden fare, such as fried foods. That way, you can eat bigger portions. On a salad, for example, sprinkle seasonings, lemon juice, or flavored vinegar in place of a heavy dressing.

Step away from sweets and salt. I rarely crave sweets, salty foods, or junk food, since I wasn't brought up with them. I never keep them in the house because when I don't have them around, I don't miss them. Skip them for a while and then take a bite. You'll see what I mean. Start by replacing cakes and cookies with fresh fruit. Scrape some salt off crackers or pretzels or buy low-salt versions. And keep in mind this saying the next time you look at that piece of chocolate (or ice cream or cake): 10 seconds in the mouth, a few hours in the stomach, a lifetime on the hips.

Get Going with Grete

Here are some easy ways to burn extra calories.

- ⮑ Add a walk, a game of catch, or some other physical activity to your evening schedule. It has been shown that as little as 10 minutes of physical activity in the evening can increase your metabolic rate.
- ⮑ Do as the Europeans do: Eat your main meal at lunch and have a lighter supper.

Drink plenty of fluids. By fluids I mean water and other nonsugary, noncaffeinated drinks. Sometimes the body is signaling thirst, not hunger. Fluids also can help fill your stomach so you don't overeat. It's best to drink 8 to 10 glasses of water a day. Remember to take in more fluids if you exercise. Take along plastic drink bottles wherever you go. If plain water is unappealing, flavor it with a small amount of fruit juice or lemon.

Eat when you're hungry; stop when you're satisfied. It takes your brain about 20 minutes to get the message that your body has been fed. Sometimes it may take a bit longer, so give the message plenty of time to kick in. Don't eat until you feel very full. This causes you to overeat and gain weight. Pay attention to your portion sizes and figure out how much fills you up. I'm aware of the proper meal size for me. If I eat my normal portion and want more, I wait 20 minutes. After that time passes, I'm often not hungry. This technique also might help you cut down on desserts.

Avoid long spells of abstinence. Abstinence will just make you ravenous later, causing you to overeat and probably to eat the wrong foods. In the long term, it slows down your metabolism. This happens because you drop below your set point (the number of calories your body is programmed to need). When you dip below your set point, your body protects itself by drastically slowing its calorie burning.

Eat regularly, not chaotically. When it comes to distribution of your meals, think of your body as a furnace. If you feed it often, it burns well. If you put all your fuel in at once, it gets very warm but only for a short time, then it gets cold again, so spread out your eating over the day. Eat at least a light breakfast, even if it's only a blender yogurt drink. Make midday eating convenient, or carry a sandwich, fruit, carrots, or crackers with you if you feel too rushed to stop for lunch. Many people make the classic mistake of skipping breakfast (there's little time, and it's usually the least social meal), having a light lunch, and eating the bulk of their food in the evening, when the body is shutting down and doesn't need the fuel.

When I was competing in southern Europe, specifically Italy and Spain, I found that dinner is traditionally eaten very late and restaurants often don't open until 7:30 P.M. I felt uncomfortable eating so late, especially because I went to bed early, so I ended up buying food to make myself an earlier meal.

According to a study of American women's diets, the average woman consumes almost half her daily calories between dinner and bedtime. Because evening snacks are often less nutritious, the same study found that these women get less vitamin C, vitamin B_6, and folic acid and more fat. Also, some scientists theorize that waiting to consume calories later in the day may contribute to weight problems by setting people up to binge. People may view bingeing as a reward for starving themselves during the day.

Keep It Simple

In recent years, studies have focused on what type of energy, or fuel, is burned by different exercises. One theory is that strenuous or all-out exercise forces the body to burn more readily available carbohydrates for energy and thus burn less fat. Therefore, you will burn more fat (and lose more weight) if you exercise slowly and steadily. If there is a difference in what a person burns, I think it's negligible. When we exercise, we burn calories. A calorie is a calorie. No matter what exercise you choose, the important thing is to do it consistently.

Exercising more slowly to burn more fat has been used as a justification to prescribe exercising longer and more gradually. I believe this theory became popular to justify slowing down and making exercise more comfortable. If exercisers, specifically beginners, push too hard, they won't stay with an exercise program. The feeling of a pounding heart and being out of breath can be very intimidating. For someone to stick with an exercise, it has to feel comfortable and safe. Exercising regularly is the goal. If moderate exercise is the best way to ensure safety and consistency, that's fine.

The harder your body works, the more fuel (calories) it requires. The math is simple: If you work out for 40 minutes at an easy pace, you will burn calories, but you will burn more of them if you work out more intensely for those same 40 minutes.

I've experimented with my own training. I've calculated that by walking 6 miles, taking into consideration my pace and body weight, I burn 450 calories. Running the same distance at a comfortable pace, I burn 550 calories. The difference in calories isn't much, but the difference in time and effort is great. The walk takes a lot longer—almost twice as long as the run. This is not to negate the benefits of walking. It is an excellent activity for sedentary people to get moving and to lose weight and build fitness.

I believe it is easier and more accurate to consider simple calorie burning than to base your exercise on whether it burns carbohydrates or fat. By burning enough calories, you'll realize the weight loss you desire.

Accept Who You Are

Body size and build are greatly determined by genetics. If you have an ideal body in mind, you have to balance that vision by accepting your body type. For example, if you have stocky legs, you're never going to have the body of Cindy Crawford—no matter how much you work out or what you eat.

On the other hand, although your body type was given to you at birth, for the most part you can fashion the flesh and muscles that hang on it.

Even six years after retiring from competitive running, I still have the look of a long-distance runner. I enjoy running and working out, and these activities help me to keep my athletic look. I accept my body as it is, which is quite slim. I realize that typical female curves will never be a part of my shape.

Many people have an unrealistic vision of how they want to look. They believe that losing weight will make them happy and healthy. That isn't necessarily true. For both the beginning exerciser and the elite athlete, the bathroom scale is only part of the health and fitness equation. Being thinner doesn't automatically make a person healthy or emotionally fulfilled, and it doesn't always make a better athlete.

It is important to have a balanced, sensible perspective on your body. Do you really need that thin, supposedly athletic look? Every time I go to the gym, I see women working out at a good pace and lifting weights. Many of them would not be considered skinny, but they're clearly in good shape. We tend to see being thin as being fit and healthy. But you can be 5 to 10 pounds overweight and still be healthy. Those few pounds are cosmetic, not a threat to your health or fitness.

The Body's Feel-Good Chemicals

For years I have been asked the same question in running clinics: "Do you experience runner's high?" I don't know a single serious or elite runner who has ever claimed to feel runner's high. While I'm running hard, I'm focused on the intensity of my effort. On easy or recovery runs, I don't feel high, or outside my body. In general, I typically feel a combination of fatigue and pleasure derived from my accomplishment, not a druglike elation.

It is said that runner's high is caused by an increase in endorphins, a chemical produced by the pituitary gland. Endorphins and morphine are similar in makeup, which creates the association of a druglike state and the idea of gaining pleasure from, or even feeling an addiction to, exercise. But the endorphin-exercise connection is still largely speculative. A relationship between long-distance running and elevated endorphins has not been clearly established. Some experts have speculated that a certain type of personality or environment makes some people susceptible to runner's high and the resistance to pain that seems to go along with it.

Studies have shown that some people's endorphins don't increase with exercise, while others' do. The perception of the endorphin effect also is very individual. It is still a mystery to researchers why some people feel runner's high during exercise, some after exercise, and some not at all.

Research has shown that the more intense the exercise, the greater the elevation of endorphins. However, you would probably need to exercise very intensely to ensure the release of a significant amount of endorphins.

David T. Lowenthal, M.D., Ph.D., is an experienced marathoner who lives near me in Gainesville, Florida. He believes that the same endorphins activated by running are triggered by any sense of achievement, from creating a satisfying piece of art or music to doing well on an exam. If you are tight or tired after running a race or training hard, or if you have a subpar performance, you probably won't feel runner's high. You might, however, feel it after a great effort.

Another factor in feeling runner's high may be the environment. You may feel different when running on a cold, rainy, miserable day than when running on a beautiful day or when surrounded by magnificent scenery.

One study concluded that runner's high should be renamed "athletic calm." A sense of athletic accomplishment and having a healthy body contribute to peace of mind. I think athletic calm is a more accurate description of what people call runner's high.

For me, the act of training, working the muscles, has a positive impact on my mood. I always feel better and more energized after exercising. There are tangible benefits to being in good shape. With a strong heart and well-toned muscles, the body functions at a higher level. I have the energy and strength to live a more vital everyday life. But you don't have to be an elite athlete to get that feeling. Many of my friends who work out feel the same way, and they've never been athletes.

When you are fit, you can take your feeling of well-being a step further. I tell the athletes I coach to imagine this scenario when training: You are running at a good clip but comfortably enough to pick up the pace—to stride out (sprint). You're up on your toes; your arms are pumping; you feel as if you're floating and you're as powerful as a gazelle. You are running quickly but under control. I use this image with my athletes in order to help them feel the power they need to excel in a race.

Workout Fundamentals
Doing Things Right from the Start

When I conduct my fitness clinics, I describe a scenario to the audience and ask them to choose between one of two outcomes. The scenario involves a decision made in early adulthood concerning one's lifestyle for the next 50 years.

The first choice is a life of leisure, but also of bad habits. It involves a lot of lounging around with minimal exercise, eating junk food and sweets, and possibly heavy drinking and smoking. Maybe you'd have a good time for all those years, but by age 70, if you made it that far, you'd probably be weak, sickly, and bedridden.

The second option is a life of activity and good habits. This life is filled with frequent exercise and a diet consisting of a lot of fruits and vegetables and very few fats. There might be some drinking, but only in moderation. At age 70, you would probably be a vital, active person and have no problem keeping up with your grandchildren.

I then ask the audience which person they'd like to be at age 70. Of course, everyone wants to be healthy and active. Here are some lifestyle questions to help you gauge which outcome you may be headed for in your later years.

↪ Do you normally take the elevator instead of the stairs?

↪ Do you always drive to destinations that are within walking distance?

↪ Is your idea of physical activity sitting on the couch and using the remote control to channel surf?

↪ Were you in better shape two years ago?

↪ Do you look less and less like your passport or driver's license photo?

↪ Have your pants really shrunk in the washing machine or have you expanded beyond the waistband's ability to meet your increasing needs?

↪ Do your exercise clothes seldom need washing?

↪ Is it increasingly difficult to tie your shoelaces?

↪ Do you feel as if you've run a marathon after walking up a flight of stairs?

↪ Do you smoke?

↪ Is it hard to refuse a gooey dessert?

↪ Do you feel as if you don't have any energy?

If you answered yes to any of these questions, you could use a workout program. If this list closely resembles your life, you need a user-friendly program—the type that takes into consideration the average American lifestyle.

Getting Started

This chapter includes my beginning walking-to-running program. The reason I chose these two activities is that they are so easy. You can do them anytime, anywhere, and you don't need any fancy equipment. All you need is a good pair of shoes.

I have prescribed this program, which I began using in 1990, to thousands of people. They have ranged in age from the late twenties to the early sixties and include groups such as the Women's Seniors Association and Manpower (the employment agency) in Norway, various corporations in the United States, and women who run the Advil Mini-Marathon in New York City. Many of the 45,000 women who participate in the Grete Waitz Run in Oslo use it. All these people can't be wrong.

The goal of the program is to work up to jogging 3 miles at a time. The more general goal is to get stronger and fitter. Many people express disappointment when they begin this program. They feel that it is too slow and gradual. "Why aren't I more tired? Why aren't I breathing hard and sweating?" they ask me. The reason the program starts slowly is that in the beginning, your body needs to adjust. For the first few weeks, you have to get your wheels moving—get the muscles, ligaments, and joints

Get Going with Grete

If the extent of your exercise over the past year has been to walk from the parking lot to your workplace, you need to start your exercise program gradually. Begin by exercising for 15 to 20 minutes three times a week, at an intensity that causes you to breathe hard and break out in a sweat. Don't push yourself to the point where you can't hold a conversation. Some great activities to start with include jogging, swimming, tennis, squash, cross-country skiing, and even heavy gardening. Give yourself 3 to 5 minutes on both ends of the workout to warm up and cool down. Within four to six weeks, you should increase your workout to at least 30 minutes three to five times a week.

in gear. The idea that all exercise has to make you breathe hard and sweat is a myth. I tell beginners doing this program that if they want that kind of workout, they should talk to me in two months.

The goal of a beginning exercise program should be to get you fit and to make you feel safe and comfortable. When asked about a typical case history, I always bring up my mother. She started exercising relatively late in life and needed to feel secure as a beginner. This program fit her needs perfectly and has since been important to her on many levels. One benefit that we could not have foreseen was that an exercise program helped her cope with becoming a widow.

The more knowledge I gained over the years about health and fitness, the more concerned I became about my sedentary parents. Unfortunately, my dad was a hopeless case. He didn't even run to catch the bus. In 1989, I handed my mother her first sweatsuit and running shoes. "I have a race of 45,000 women," I told her, "and you have to be part of it." At first she presented me with all the obstacles, including the fact that she was 65 years old. I responded by making her an offer

(continued on page 42)

Walking-to-Running Program

	Day 1	Day 2	Day 3
Week 1	Walk 5 min. Jog 1 min./walk 1 min. x 6 Walk 5 min. 22 min. total	Walk 5 min. Jog 1 min./walk 1 min. x 7 Walk 5 min. 24 min. total	Same as Day 2 24 min. total
Week 2	Walk 5 min. Jog 1 min./walk 1 min. x 4 Jog 2 min./walk 2 min. x 2 Jog 1 min./walk 1 min. x 2 25 min. total	Same as Day 1 25 min. total	Same as Day 1 25 min. total
Week 3	Walk 5 min. Jog 2 min./walk 2 min. x 2 Jog 3 min./walk 3 min. x 2 Jog 4 min. Walk 2 min. 31 min. total	Same as Day 1 31 min. total	Same as Day 1 31 min. total
Week 4	Walk 5 min. Jog 5 min. Walk 3 min. Jog 7 min. Walk 5 min. Jog 5 min. Walk 4 min. 34 min. total	Walk 5 min. Jog 6 min. Walk 3 min. Jog 6 min. Walk 3 min. Jog 4 min. Walk 3 min. 30 min. total	Same as Day 2 30 min. total
Week 5	Walk 5 min. Jog 4 min./walk 1 min. x 2 Jog 8 min. Walk 2 min. Jog 6 min. Walk 2 min. 33 min. total	Walk 5 min. Jog 7 min. Walk 2 min. Jog 5 min./walk 1 min. x 2 Jog 8 min. Walk 2 min. 36 min. total	Same as Day 1 33 min. total

Day 1	Day 2	Day 3
Week 6 Walk 5 min. Jog 7 min./walk 2 min. x 2 Jog 8 min. Walk 2 min. Jog 3 min. Walk 2 min. 38 min. total 36 min. total	Walk 5 min. Jog 10 min. Walk 3 min. Jog 8 min. Walk 2 min. Jog 6 min. Walk 2 min.	Same as Day 1 38 min. total
Week 7 Walk 5 min. Jog 12 min. Walk 2 min. Jog 8 min./walk 1 min. x 2 37 min. total	Same as Day 1 37 min. total	Same as Day 1 37 min. total
Week 8 Walk 5 min. Jog 15 min. Walk 2 min. Jog 15 min. Walk 3 min. 40 min. total	Same as Day 1 40 min. total	Same as Day 1 40 min. total
Week 9 Walk 5 min. Jog 20 min. Walk 2 min. Jog 10 min. Walk 3 min. 40 min. total	Same as Day 1 40 min. total	Same as Day 1 40 min. total
Week 10 Walk 5 min. Jog 30 min. Walk 5 min. 40 min. total	Same as Day 1 40 min. total	Same as Day 1 40 min. total

What Is a Workout?

↳ A workout is not just an exercise session. It is part of a lifestyle.

↳ It consists of 75 percent willpower and discipline and 25 percent perspiration.

↳ It makes you better than you were yesterday.

↳ It is a victory over laziness and coming up with bad excuses.

↳ It increases your self-confidence.

↳ It makes you feel good about yourself.

she couldn't refuse: I would train with her.

The race, which is 5 kilometers, or 3.1 miles, takes place in May, and we began training in February. We started by walking 1 mile three times a week. When she could walk 2 miles at a time, I introduced a bit of running. "Now we'll jog to the next light pole," I instructed. I listened carefully to her breathing and monitored her heart rate. (It is important to increase exercise slowly and not to overtrain.) In six to seven weeks, she began training by herself.

On race day, my mother crossed the finish line in 38 minutes, a very respectable time for someone who had been training for only about four months. She's done the event four times since, and now she swims twice a week and takes long walks. She's proud of herself, and I'm proud of her, too. Recently, after taking a long hike, she said, "Now I'm going to sit down and not move." I told her it's better to be tired this way than to be tired from doing nothing all day.

Two Different Things

Throughout this book, I use the terms health and fitness together, but technically they are not one and the same. Health refers to a person's entire profile: fitness level, exercise and nutrition habits, and overall physical and mental wellness. You can't objectively measure optimum health, but you can measure fitness. Doctors and professionals most commonly measure fitness by calculating VO_2 max, the maximum volume of oxygen your body consumes during exertion. More informally, you can measure your fitness by running a 5-K race or swimming laps for time.

Being fit doesn't necessarily mean being healthy. I meet a lot of people who believe they are healthy just because they run. But if their diet is poor, they drink alcohol excessively, or they are under significant and continual stress, they are probably not healthy. Too many of these people believe that they can get away with anything because they work out.

This is also true of some world-class athletes, specifically those using illegal substances in hopes of enhancing their performance. In my competitive days, anabolic steroids were the most popular performance-enhancing drugs. Women who used them sometimes had deeper voices or more facial hair. I also heard about football players and weight lifters who contracted cancer because of steroids. I would never do anything to jeopardize my health. I knew that the occasional cortisone shot to alleviate an injury was not illegal, but I wanted to make sure it wasn't unhealthy either. I agreed to take these shots only after I was certain that they would not compromise my health.

Clearly, athletes with specific race or training goals cannot achieve those goals merely by maintaining health. But they can't get the most out of themselves without good health. The best recommendation I can make to the average person is to develop and maintain optimal health and basic fitness. That is why I provide both training and lifestyle advice in this book. If you exercise on a regular basis, eat well, live sensibly, and maintain a sense of humor, you will create the balance that helps maintain health and fitness.

Figuring Out Fitness

When you go on a car trip, it helps to know how to reach your destination. But before you can figure that out, you need to know where you're starting from. The same goes for building fitness. To set realistic goals and work out appropriately, you need to know your fitness level and what kind of exerciser you are.

As I mentioned previously, aerobic fitness can be measured by calculating your VO_2 max. But this is not a practical suggestion for the average person. Unless you're a professional athlete who can benefit by this exact measurement, there's no need to go through the testing. More reasonably, total fitness can be broken down into five categories: cardiorespiratory, strength, muscular endurance, flexibility, and body composition. By determining your starting level in these areas, you can see how fit you are and tailor your exercise program appropriately.

Cardiorespiratory. Also known as *aerobic* or *cardiovascular* fitness. These terms generally refer to the same thing: the body's ability to generate energy for working muscles during sustained exercise. More than anything else, this depends on the efficient delivery of oxygen from the heart and lungs. The more efficient your body is at delivering oxygen to your cells, the fitter you are. Sustained-effort activities such as running, swimming, biking, and cross-country skiing will improve your cardiorespiratory fitness. Studies have shown that the ideal amount of sustained-effort exercise for optimum cardiovascular fitness is 20 to 30 minutes three times a week, done at a moderate level of intensity. Because my sport is running and I have developed running and walking programs, I base the following cardiorespiratory fitness levels on these activities.

Beginner. You fall into this category if you have walked at a moderate pace for 20 to 30 minutes three times a week for several months. Although this activity is not very taxing, it is aerobic.

Intermediate. This is someone who can complete 2 miles at a pace of 15 minutes per mile by fast walking, jogging, or a combination of the two three times a week.

Serious. A very aerobically fit person can do half an hour of continuous jogging at a pace of 10 minutes per mile or faster three times a week.

Strength, muscular endurance, and flexibility. Strength and muscular endurance are measured by how much weight you can lift and how many times you can lift that weight. Flexibility refers to whether or not you can put your muscles through their full range of motion. Why is that important? Because muscles get more powerful only within the range in which they're used. Exercising with tight muscles will shortchange your workout. The stretching (for flexibility) and strengthening (for muscular strength and endurance) exercises in chapter 8 can be used to gauge your fitness level in these areas. If you can't complete at least one set of an exercise, you are a beginner. If you can complete one or two sets, you're at an intermediate level. And if you can perform all sets of an exercise, you are at the optimal fitness level in these categories.

Fast Fitness

How do you know if you're getting a workout? You can keep track of your heart rate, but in time, experience will tell you when you are in "the zone." I know when I'm taxed and when an activity isn't working for me. When everyone raved about how fun aerobics classes were, I decided to give one a try. It looked easy, but I was terrible at it. As soon as I caught on to one exercise, the instructor moved on to another. I didn't break a sweat, and I wasn't breathing hard. If you pick a sport that requires some skill, such as tennis, squash, or aerobics, concentrate on developing that skill so that you'll get a worthwhile workout.

Body composition. As a rule, fitness improves when the body has more muscle and less fat. There are various ways to measure your percentage of body fat: calipers that measure skin folds at different sites on the body, underwater weighing (very accurate but highly impractical), and home body fat monitors and scales. The Tanita Corporation of America is one company that makes a variety of home monitors and scales. For further information, call 1-800-TANITA-8.

My favorite measure is the waistband test. I have one pair of jeans I use to measure my body composition. If they fit around the waist, I am at my optimal weight. If they are too tight, I know I have gained a few pounds. I think the common adage about body composition is a good one: Don't use the scale; just look at how your clothes fit.

Exercisers Are Not All Alike

I believe that exercisers differ in one major aspect: intention. Approaching a workout as an enjoyable, beneficial activity instead of a burdensome chore is much more important than possessing athletic ability. There are, however, other, more concrete characteristics of the different levels of exercisers.

Beginner. A sporadic exerciser, such as an occasional walker, or someone beginning a new activity. (An experienced walker is not a beginner, but a walker undertaking a jogging program is.) A beginner exercises somewhat regularly (two to four times a week), but missing a week is not uncommon.

The goal of the beginner is to go from a sedentary to a more active lifestyle. At this level, he isn't training for the Olympics, or even for competition. The point is to experience the satisfaction and benefits of physical activity. I often meet people who tell me that they don't enjoy exercise that much, but they like what it does for them—for their body, mind, and mood.

Intermediate. Someone who works out four or five times per week. This exerciser may enjoy training for races, for example, but would probably not increase training to become more competitive. Although exercise is a priority, it is not *the* priority. An intermediate exerciser would not rearrange his life to accommodate exercise.

The training program in this chapter moves the beginner up to the level of jogging slowly for 5 kilometers (3.1 miles). Many of those who use the program move ahead, running up to 4 miles at a time. Then they decide that they would like to participate in a race or perhaps run faster. Good examples of intermediate exercisers are most of the 150,000 participants in the Chase Corporate Challenge. A variety of factors can motivate people at this level. As they improve, they realize that they can do better. They watch a race or other activity and are inspired to try it. They get a taste of success and want to have more of it.

Serious. Someone who works out six or seven days a week and sometimes may work out twice in one day. The serious exerciser probably spends an hour or more each day working out and may have a double routine (running, swimming, or cycling as the main sport, plus a weight program).

There is a clear difference between beginner and intermediate, but a finer line between intermediate and serious. (There's also a clear difference between serious and national or world-class. Being a world-class athlete is a full-time job.) I use the term *serious*, as opposed to *advanced*, because *serious* reflects intention more than ability. Intermediate exercisers try to maximize the time they spend training—to squeeze out of it what they can. Serious exercisers adjust their lifestyle in some manner to accommodate training. You can be a 4-hour

Tips from the Top

As you become fitter, you'll need to increase the intensity of your exercise from time to time. As your body adapts, you won't have to work as hard to achieve the same results, but you'll need to work harder to continue to gain strength. To avoid boredom as you increase your exercise, consider changing your activity. Try running fartlek (varying your pace for random distances) or intervals (varying the pace—speeding up, then slowing down to recover—for set distances), jumping rope, biking, or swimming.

marathoner and still be serious—if you have made certain sacrifices or changes in your job or family life to train.

You must consider your personality type and lifestyle when evaluating which level of exerciser you are or are considering becoming. In striving for a higher level, you must consider whether you can tolerate the added physical and emotional stress from increased training. It will do you no good, nor will you see any improvement, if you take on more than you can handle. And you'll also risk injuring yourself.

Too Much of a Good Thing

The fitness industry spends a great deal of time and money to get people to start exercising, but very little attention is paid to the other side of the coin: overtraining. Perhaps it would be more accurate to call this practice over*straining*. From my experience, less serious exercisers often associate overtraining with world-class athletes. But it doesn't just happen to the professionals. Even exercising three times a week can be too much if it is more than your body or lifestyle can tolerate. Also, at any level, too much too soon can be overtraining.

Overtraining can be a tricky condition to diagnose. Two of the

Tips from the Top

Here are some ways to keep from pushing too hard with your exercise.

Don't punish yourself. Exercise should not be used to make amends if you stumble in other areas of your life. If you stray from good eating habits, for example, don't overexert yourself just to make up for it.

Preparation is key. Just as you get mentally ready to train, get ready for a rest. Pick a day, vow to take it off, and then do it.

Think positive thoughts. Convince yourself that rest is good for you and that you don't want to be addicted to exercise.

Observe what happens on rest days. Nothing changes—not your life, not the world. This will help calm you, and when you experience better training after a break, you will realize that you are doing what is best for you.

symptoms are staleness and fatigue. Here are some other signs that could indicate you're overdoing it and you should probably scale back on your exercising.

- Persistent soreness that doesn't go away after you have warmed up
- Minor aches and pains that don't go away
- Frequent sore throats, colds, or other illnesses
- Uncharacteristic short-temperedness or irritability
- Insomnia or loss of appetite

For most people, over-training is a result of exercise plus the stress of everyday life. When I was training for the 1984 Olympics, I became overextended by having to take on added responsibilities during a family crisis. It wasn't until I felt run-down and out of energy and my performances became flat that I realized I had to scale back and get others to pitch in to help.

At Vidar, my sports club in Norway, not all the runners are serious. Most have jobs or are students. All have busy lives. When they ask me for advice, it is usually because something has gone wrong in their training. I ask them how things are going in their lives in general. That is usually how I discover the roots of their problems. Some of the runners are training like top-class athletes but can't live like professionals. Professionals have state-of-the-art medical care, nutrition, massage, and a minimum of outside distractions. Many of the people who consult me swear that they don't train hard, but if training is interfering with their lives to the point where problems are cropping up, it's too much.

On the opposite end of the spectrum is the balanced life of my 53-year-old brother Jan. He is a hard worker who co-owns his business, has two grown sons who are independent, and is a determined, ordered, optimistic, and relaxed person. He also has years of sports experience, a genetic gift, and a best marathon time of 2:29. When he decides to run the New York City Marathon, he knows that our brother Arild is going to take charge of their business; his training has been done at home, and there is nothing he can do to change that once he's in New York; worrying will not help; and he is going to have a good time in the Big Apple. Unlike so many other runners, he doesn't get distracted by last-minute gimmicks such as special diets or running aids. My brother's inner self is calm, stable, and confident. As a result, he has run 16 marathons under 3 hours, most recently a 2:58.

I meet all kinds of people and all kinds of exercisers. Some are overstressed and obsessed. Others are like my brother Jan, who runs a marathon after an evening out on the town. The beauty of sports and exercise is that not only are you forced to consider the type of person you are before you choose a routine, but these activities also help you to see exactly who you are and what you are made of. Often one of the great discoveries people make about themselves is that they are tougher, smarter, and more resilient than they thought they were.

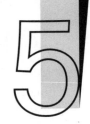

It's All in the Mind
The Psychological Benefits of Exercise

We all have different motivations for exercising: our own well-being, socializing with friends, a doctor's advice. I believe people work out mostly for their own well-being, with a minority motivated by the social aspect or a doctor's prescription. I'm the opposite of a person who seeks a social experience. Maybe you could say I am the classic long-distance runner. I like my solitude. In fact, I am not very social at all in my exercise. With the exception of some training runs with my husband or brother Jan (and I emphasize that they were mostly silent runs), I have never chatted while running. Even today, in retirement, I find it very distracting if there is conversation during a run.

I work out as much for my head as I do for my body. I'm a thinker. A lot of my ideas come to me more easily when I am running. That is why I like to run in the morning, when there are no distractions such as people and traffic. That isn't the way it was when I was competing. Then, almost every run had a purpose, a goal. I focused primarily on the running. Now, some of my best ideas are born on the run.

Sometimes our lives are like balloons, just waiting to burst. Stress keeps building up, and there seems to be no way to vent it. Many years ago, people expended a lot more physical energy. That helped keep a balance between the mental and physical parts of their lives. If you exercise, even sporadically, you know how great it is for letting off steam. Even before I was conscious of using exercise for stress reduction, I was in fact using it that way. In my student days, when the work was very stressful, I always felt better after running. I didn't know it at the time, but now I realize that it helped me cope with, and excel in, my studies.

Be Secure and Confident

In my exercise program, and my general philosophy, I stress the doable. I want people to feel secure and open to success. I know that the difficulty getting started involves more than getting motivated. Part of it may be the fear of being observed and judged. That may have been prevalent 15 years ago, but today when you look at exercisers, you see all shapes and sizes. People aren't as judgmental anymore; they know that everyone should get in shape. I admire the people who are out there making the effort. It's great that they're taking charge of their lives and want to get in shape. Even my mother, at age 65, wasn't shy about running. She knew other women her age who were doing it, and I was very supportive, making sure she felt comfortable at all times— emotionally as well as physically.

Despite this general change in attitude, the fear of being judged harshly remains for many exercisers. If you are feeling shy about working out, these tips can help.

Choose mass-participation events. Road races, walkathons, and bike-a-thons are great events where you can blend into the crowd. The more participants there are, the better. They provide a protective shield for those who are feeling insecure.

Dress like the rest. There's no need to buy expensive outfits or equipment to work out. With shorts and a T-shirt or a sweatsuit, you'll fit right in.

Enlist your friends. Being among people you're comfortable with goes a long way toward helping you overcome your shyness. You also can join a group or club of beginning exercisers. Inquire at a local gym, fitness center, or running or walking club about these groups.

Go it alone. If you'd rather train by yourself, pick isolated places or times of the day when others usually don't train. Remember, however, to take extra safety precautions if you train alone.

Stay at home. The abundance of excellent exercise videos and moderately priced home exercise equipment makes it very easy to get a great workout without ever stepping outside your house.

Seek out the pros. Being shy often comes from being intimidated by lack of knowledge. Educate yourself about the activity you're interested in, and your confidence will grow.

Take inspiration from others. Keep in mind that many people have changed their lives for the better because of exercise. If they can do it, you can, too.

Ever notice the glow of an exerciser or the look of joy on a racer's face as he crosses the finish line and punches his fist into the air in triumph? Exercise gives us an enormous sense of satisfaction and confidence. This becomes apparent when I work with women for my yearly race in Norway, the Grete Waitz Run. Women have come up to me and said, "When I finished the race, I knew I could do a lot more in my life." I received a letter from a woman who said running had changed her life. She was more secure, independent, and happy, and she was able to get out of a bad marriage. These women went from seeing themselves as nonathletes to seeing themselves as being able to conquer the world.

The most stunning example I know of the positive mental impact of exercise comes from a three-month pilot fitness program I conducted. It was sponsored by the Norwegian government for the unemployed, a group with very low self-esteem and self-confidence. The sense of failure these people felt in their work lives spread to their personal lives. They believed that getting in shape and quitting smoking were unobtainable goals. The first time they walked into the gym, they looked defeated, as if they had the weight of the world on their shoulders.

The program included exercise and lessons on anatomy and how to train. When the participants realized they could, and did, get in better shape, they felt like winners. Midway through the program, they began to come into the gym with smiles on their faces. They said they had something to wake up for each morning. Many seriously considered giving up smoking. And they even decided, entirely on their own, to enter a 5-K race.

At the end of the program, participants could take an optional test if they wanted to lead future beginning exercise groups. Seventy-five percent of the people passed the test. They were amazed at their achievements. I was surprised to see that even the ones I thought were shy and reserved were willing to lead groups. The success they achieved in their exercise programs spilled over into other areas of their lives. They became motivated to seek employment or take a re-training course.

The Power of Visualization

Exercise and sports are greatly affected by what goes on in the mind, and the mind is greatly affected by exercise and sports as well. This is true among exercisers at all levels, despite their different goals.

I mention goals because without them, it is difficult to use your mental powers to fuel what you do. First, you have to decide what you want to get out of your training. It's particularly important for beginners to make sure their aspirations are obtainable.

When you have set a realistic and specific goal, you can move to the next step: mental training. A major element in mental training is visualization. No complex skills are needed to master this technique. I believe it comes naturally to most people. Whether planning your career or imagining your unborn baby, you have probably done it. Visualizing a positive outcome can create a pattern of success, as long as you set realistic and specific goals.

In my running career, visualization always came with very little mental effort. When I trained, I had a specific scene in my mind: being on the starting line, running a specific race, and finishing number one. When visualization was a hot topic in the 1980s, people would approach me and ask about my mental preparation. I didn't know what they meant. Then I read about visualization and realized that I had been doing it ever since my teens.

To become adept at visualization, you must practice focusing on your exercise. Often you may use a run or time at the gym to daydream, compose your day's schedule, or think through a problem. That's fine occasionally, but try to get in the habit of being in the present. Talk to yourself about your exercise; convince yourself of success and of the likelihood of achieving your goal. See events in detail: the place, the time, the way you look and move.

Don't reserve visualization just for training time. When I was competing, I could be driving or reading a book, and my mind would be in the New York City Marathon. I didn't *decide* to think of the race; it would just pop into my head. And when I would think about winning, my heart rate would go up. I could physically feel the rush of success as a powerful effect of visualization.

I have brought the same visualization and focus to other aspects of my life. Before I give a speech or do a clinic, I go over the events in my mind. Whether I'm negotiating a deal or trying to resolve a personal relationship, this technique carries over from my exercise.

Training Smarts

Most fitness books and training programs concentrate on motivating people to do something: to walk farther, run faster, or get stronger. Although doing is very important, we all need to be able *not* to do.

Pushing ourselves often becomes a symbol of our discipline and toughness. But these good habits also can lead to overtraining and an obsession with exercise.

I tell the athletes I coach that it takes guts to train hard and push yourself, but it also takes guts, and a lot of self-confidence, to back off when necessary. The most successful exercisers or athletes are more than just the most disciplined, the most dedicated, or the toughest. They also are the smartest. They back off and rest when they know they should. The most consistent and enduring athletes are almost always the ones with the most sensible training programs. But backing off isn't easy for many of us. We think that doing so means that we have no guts or that we're getting soft.

If I could go back and do anything differently in my career, it would be to rest more. I was so competitive that I trained relentlessly. Even when I knew I would be better off resting more, I went out and trained. I always thought that my competitors were doing that and I had to be even tougher. There were no heart rate monitors or instant blood evaluations when I was competing. I rested only when the doctor gave me a blood test, saw that I was not recovering properly, and told me to cut back on my training.

Now I tell my athletes, many of whom push themselves relentlessly, that they shouldn't make the same mistakes I made 15 years ago. I tell them that addiction to training is not really about problematic exercise; it's about a problematic life.

Sensible exercise is not just good for you; it also leads to success and satisfaction. When athletes on any level train intelligently, they get tangible results such as fast race times and victories. That gives them the self-confidence and sense of security they need to continue striving for success. It opens the door to other good things in their lives. They are more relaxed and happier with themselves, and other people like them better, too.

My co-author, Gloria Averbuch, is a good example of the positive outcome of "training smarts." We were chatting on the phone one Saturday morning several years ago. She told me she was a bit tense, which was characteristic of her mood until she did her daily workout. In the course of the conversation, she admitted to once seeing her hands begin to shake after going for several days without exercise.

On that particular morning, she was tired and unmotivated to run. "So don't run," I told her. "Go out and take a walk with your children." She laughed, and although it took her a while to be convinced, she vowed to try it. She called me back a few days later to thank me. Not only did she have the energy and strength to go for a nice, long walk with her daughters, but she felt that her fitness had made it possible to chase and play with them so effortlessly. What's more, the following day she was well rested and had a great run. The rest day led to an exciting and joyful revelation. She had spent many years working out, but she had rarely taken the time to stop and smell the roses.

Total Fitness

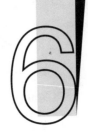

Running and Walking
The Road to Success

You'll hear a lot of running and walking advice over time. I have. And even though I am about to give you some more advice based on my years of experience, I want to start with this essential point: It's not the speed at which you run, where you run, or when you run that counts. Going out and doing it is most important. The tips in this chapter are meant to be helpful and educational, but don't let the information distract you from the act of putting one foot in front of the other.

An Ideal Exercise

Running provides the same cardiorespiratory benefits as aerobic exercise, but it has some additional advantages as well, especially for busy people.

> ↳ Running is versatile. That's why it's the ideal exercise for those with a limited amount of time. You can do it anywhere, anytime, or with anyone. Running doesn't require special facilities, sophisticated equipment, a lot of money, or a partner. All you need is a good pair of shoes.

- You don't need special training or special skills to run. It's probably the only exercise that you used to do regularly (as a child) but that, at some point, you stopped doing.
- Running offers something for all ages. Road races are proof of this. People from 2 to 90 participate in these events.
- Next to cross-country skiing, running burns more calories than any other aerobic activity. It takes a lot more energy to carry your body weight than it does to work out sitting down, as on a bicycle or rowing machine.
- Running is a perfect activity for those who travel a lot or are on the go. A good run in these circumstances not only keeps you fit but also helps keep you relaxed and better able to handle your schedule.
- Running is the basis for other sports and activities, such as soccer and tennis. When I took up cross-country ski competition for a time, I was successful because of my fitness base from running.
- Running is an excellent endurance conditioner for everything from dancing to the rigors of daily life—whether climbing stairs, lugging groceries, or keeping up with the kids.
- Running can be a social sport, or it can provide solitude and contemplation—which is how I like it. I meet people all the time who testify how running has changed their lives. They tell me how much healthier and more energetic they feel.

Among the many new runners I have counseled is a television entertainer in Norway. He was once quite overweight and is also asthmatic. I worked with him over a two-year period, which culminated in his completing the New York City Marathon. He told me that he likes how running makes him feel and what it does for him. Because of running, he lost weight, could cut back on his asthma medication, and feels more creative professionally.

My Running Life

I love running. It's as simple as that. I have devoted most of my life to running, and it has given me endless rewards: physical, emotional, and professional. The benefits of running are lifelong. I ran as a child, and I intend to run into my old age.

Over the years, I have tried to convey to people the basic ease of this activity. I don't want to complicate it. I just want people to experience the freedom of running and to have fun with it. As wonderful as my racing has been, that's not the entire story of my running. I have enjoyed running on many levels. Following are some examples of where and how I have run.

I have run all over the world—on tracks in stadiums and on the streets of major cities, but also in some unusual places. I have been very inventive in my running, especially during the 1970s, when there were no indoor treadmills and few fitness centers. For lack of space, in bad weather, or because of other reasons, I have run in airports, in parking garages, and around shopping centers. In my competitive days, during the long Norwegian winters, I trained on a 150-meter walkway down to a subway station and under a covered bus stop of the same length.

I've also run in wonderful places such as the forests of Oslo, over miles of trails and dirt paths, and on the winding roads of Bermuda; on a beach in the Canary Islands; in Japan around the Imperial Palace (the safest place in the world, as there's a guard every tenth of a mile); and on the streets of New York City, my second home, where the cabdrivers call out my name.

Running gives me a clearer perspective on the world, and it makes me feel special. I've never been a traditional tourist. I've always seen the world by running, and that has allowed me to view things in a different way. Places look different in the early-morning hours, when the streets are deserted. I've smelled crabs boiling on Fisherman's Wharf in San Francisco on my way to the Golden Gate Bridge, watched the sun rise over Diamond Head in Hawaii, and seen deer grazing on the Alps in St. Moritz, Switzerland. I clearly remember turning to my husband, Jack, in one of these places and saying, "People don't know what they're missing."

I'm very thankful that running is my primary activity for other reasons as well. It's easy to stay in shape. If I had participated in a team sport, my transition from serious training to fitness may have been more difficult. I draw tremendous psychological and emotional benefits from my running. I have a lot of energy and can handle pressure better because of running's calming effects. The constant travel that is part of my life is tough. Jet lag affects me a great deal. Finding a gym in which to work out might be difficult, but I can run almost anywhere. On my most stressful days, Jack often asks, "Why run today?" I answer that my day will be a lot more stressful if I *don't* run.

Stride and Form

Everyone knows the motion of running. You may feel out of sync or uncoordinated in the beginning, but the more you run, the more efficient you will become. Although there are guidelines, there is no one right way to run. People have different running styles, many of which may not be "by the book," but they work. People used to comment on Bill Rodgers's habit of swinging one of his arms out to the side, but it didn't affect his ability to win four Boston Marathons and four New York City Marathons. I've seen runners who look as if they're scooting along the ground, barely lifting their bodies, complete marathons in under 3 hours.

Each running distance has its classic form, although most people can't perfectly duplicate it. A sprinter's form is characterized by a forward lean. A middle-distance specialist runs with the hips forward. Marathoners, who often come from various distance backgrounds, seem to have a wider range of forms, but they generally "sit back" in the hips and run close to the ground. Although I originally ran middle distances, my running style is suited more to longer distances. I didn't have the classic forward posture of middle-distance runners such as Sebastian Coe and Mary Slaney.

I started as a 400-meter and 800-meter runner. Middle-distance runners are taught to emphasize proper form, as efficiency counts for time. To a large degree, good form is a matter of practice, but it is very difficult to achieve that form consciously. Children's running is a good illustration of this fact, since children do not deliberately concentrate on their form. When I watch children run in races, I notice that the front-runners run very efficiently and economically, while the ones farther back move their arms and legs all over the place.

Of course, there are general rules and a general style you should keep in mind. Good running form can prevent injuries and increase your efficiency and endurance. But you can't drastically alter your stride; you have to let yourself run more or less naturally. In 1980, I had a Czech coach who told me that I'd run faster if I changed my technique. I worked hard to adapt my stride. I may have been running more correctly, but I used up so much energy doing it that my times were slower.

Here are some pointers on good running form.

Watch your stride. Don't overstride or understride. If you do, you'll feel awkward and increase the likelihood of injuring yourself.

Don't run on the balls of your feet. I notice that, in particular, some women tend to run with short strides and up on their toes.

Adopt a soft touch. You can hear some runners before you see them because of the sound of their pounding. Keep your foot plant quick and light.

Focus on moving forward. This will help keep your feet and arms straight. Swing your arms back to front, not side to side, and hold them at the midpoint of your body.

Maintain good posture. Your body should be erect, not slouched over. Don't clench your fists; keep your hands loose and lightly cupped, but not flopping.

Exercise on a treadmill in front of a mirror. I do this to check my form. If this isn't possible, look in the reflection of storefront windows. Just be careful not to run into a light pole or a pedestrian.

If you are running four or more times a week, try doing some or all of the following techniques twice a week. They will help make you more aware of your body mechanics and any inefficiencies. They also will help you to run faster.

Go uphill. Hill running forces you to get stronger, work your arms more, and lift your knees higher.

Give pickups a try. Run fast without straining. Imagine that you are Carl Lewis and try to duplicate his perfect form.

Prance. Run a short distance with quick knee lifts. This strengthens the hip flexors ("levers" at the top of the legs), which aid in lifting your knees.

Practice butt kicks. Run a short distance with your heels touching your backside. This helps develop quicker leg turnover.

Relaxing and Breathing

The more you move up the steps of the ladder—the more experienced a runner you become—the more comfortable and efficient you will get. Everything will fall into place—a natural arm swing; loose, unclenched hands; and loose facial muscles—if you relax. Remember that tension takes energy. That energy is better spent on your running effort.

Faces are instructive. Look at the many top Kenyan runners. They don't grit their teeth or tighten their chins. They keep everything hanging, while rhythmically breathing through their mouths. This relaxation extends down to the neck and shoulders. The Kenyans never look strained, like some Westerners. Maybe that's because they have been running since they were very young. To them, moving forward with as little energy as possible comes naturally, which should be your goal as well. I never realized what I looked like when I ran, but I was once told I appeared to be in a trance; I never changed my facial expression.

Many runners, from beginners to those trying to push the pace in a race, ask me about breathing. Some people breathe silently; some make noises with their effort. Again, do what comes naturally. If you need to breathe audibly, do it. I've run side by side with noisy breathers and wondered how they were going to make it to the finish line, but they kept on going. Although it's okay to be a heavy breather, don't be a shallow or fast breather. Short, fast breathing also is likely to give you a side stitch, or cramp.

Overlooked Fundamentals

In much of the advice given on running, certain aspects often are not addressed. I learned some of these lessons from years of training, but I found out others by talking to people at my running clinics.

Run according to your fitness level. Very often, because of impatience, people do too much, too soon, always running on the edge of discomfort. Pushing yourself will not get you in shape more quickly, but it may get you injured. If you don't enjoy running or you are often sore or heavy-legged, slow down.

Vary your pace. Intermediate and serious runners need to do this. Runners on this level often lament that they are not improving. That's because they are running at the same comfortable pace: never easy, but also never hard. It pays to add some variety to your training. When you do this, I suggest that you use a heart rate monitor (see chapter 3) to gauge your response.

Change your routes. Avoid running the same course, the same side of a banked road, or the same direction on a track or other circular path. Varying the stress and impact will help you to avoid injury and build fitness. Try to run on different terrain—hilly as well as flat. If you run laps, alternate your direction. These changes also add variety. By reversing laps, I feel as if I am doing a different run.

Take care on hills. When running downhill, don't lean backward. Keep your body at the same angle you do while running on a flat surface. If the hill is very steep, run down zigzag or walk down. Running uphill will shorten your stride naturally, but don't forget to concentrate on your arm swing to help power you up.

Run often on surfaces such as dirt or grass. Because the impact on these surfaces is lower than on concrete, they are gentler on your legs and joints. The uneven surfaces also strengthen the ligaments around your ankles. As a veteran of cross-country running, I can testify to this.

Put treadmills to better use. If you use a treadmill, set it at a 1 to 2 percent incline. This more closely duplicates the road and gives you a better workout.

Don't fight the weather. If road conditions are bad because of rain, snow, or ice, find an alternative or take a day off. The altered running style—tightened muscles or a change in stride—required to avoid slipping or falling can cause injuries. It is also nerve-racking to run under these conditions.

Come prepared. If you plan to finish your run at a place other than home, bring a change of clothing and fluids to drink. I often drive a few miles to vary my running route. Even if it's only 10 minutes from the house, I bring fresh clothing. This helps prevent me from getting chilled and keeps my muscles from tightening up. Fluid replacement right after exercise is important to prevent dehydration.

Warm up before and cool down afterward. Do this by walking or jogging for a few hundred yards. Although I don't think this is necessary for a nontaxing, slower run, if you are really moving, you should warm up and cool down. The faster you run, the more important this is, and the longer you should take for these routines. For a good running effort, I warm up and cool down for at least half a mile.

Walking

It's the most natural physical activity there is. Everyone knows how to do it, it takes us where we want to go, and it's a great way to exercise, especially for overweight or older people. To participate, all you need is a good pair of shoes.

The majority of walkers are women. I think that men feel that walking is not macho enough. When my husband asked his business partner, an injured runner, to go walking, the man answered, "Walking—that's for old people!" But that's clearly a myth. Walking strengthens muscles, improves circulation, and burns calories. And by walking very briskly, or racewalking, you can bring your effort up to the level of an easy jog.

Walking is very versatile also—even more so than running. While in Buffalo and San Francisco, two cities I visit often for the Chase Corporate Challenge, I have seen businesspeople, even women in skirts, exercise walking along the streets during their lunch hours. Mall walking is a popular activity that I fully endorse. The mall is made available for walkers usually before store hours.

I have always used walking for exercise and pleasure. In my competitive days, when I was injured and couldn't run, I'd walk—usually an hour and a half in the woods of Oslo. I'd get my aerobic exercise on a stationary bike, but I'd keep my calf muscles working through walking.

In the early 1990s, when I had tight hamstrings and couldn't run, I used the stationary bike again, but I missed being outdoors and getting fresh air. Because the weather was so nice at my home in Gainesville, Florida, I ended up walking, which I did for an hour to an hour and a half at a brisk pace.

I still walk regularly when my schedule allows it. Although walking can't serve as exercise if you are in top shape (I've been tested walking on an inclined treadmill, and my heart rate wasn't high enough for the walk to qualify as exercise), it can serve as pleasurable recreation. Jack and I often enjoy a good, long walk as we chat and look at the scenery.

Depending on your condition, walking can contribute to fitness. If you're a normal, healthy person, your pace should be about 3½ to 4 miles per hour, and you should walk for at least 40 minutes to get a beneficial workout. You should increase your breathing and at least break into a light sweat. When you pick up the pace to make it more strenuous, use your arms to get you moving. This increased arm swing should come naturally as you move faster, but you might want to move your arms in a running motion to get the feel of how they can power you along. Also, be careful not to overstride when speeding up. It is better to move your legs at a faster rate than to lengthen your stride.

I have never done racewalking, a fast-paced, stiffer-legged walk in which the hips power the stride and the arms are used as they are in running. I've seen many racewalkers in New York City's Central Park, and it is clear that they perceive their activity as a workout, not just a stroll. Racewalking also is a competitive sport. The world-class walkers do a 10-K race in less than 40 minutes. That's a 6:30-mile pace. If racewalking interests you, search out classes or groups at walking or running clubs or at the local YMCA or YWCA.

If walking does little or nothing for you as an exercise, try speeding up or jogging lightly. Who knows, you might end up as a runner! Combination walking and jogging is very common. Most of the participants in the Grete Waitz Run are in this category. If you complete and maintain my beginning running program in chapter 4, you will be in this category, too. Keep in mind that if you choose to exercise this way, a combination of walking and running in the same session is more valuable than walking one day and running the next. If you have the ability to run for an entire session, you don't need the walking. If you're a walker, you'll get a much better aerobic workout if you add some running to your program.

If you don't walk for fitness, consider walking as something you do for health. Everyday walking, for errands or transportation, requires using the body—always a positive activity. In Norway, most people walk for transportation, especially to the train or bus stop. That's one reason you don't see many Norwegian women wearing high heels.

Walking is a great prelude to running. It uses the same basic motion and muscle groups, yet is lower impact and easier to do. For any adult past the age of 30 who has been sedentary and wants to start a running program, I always prescribe walking first. It helps to condition the joints and ligaments. In fact, the main problem I have with beginners who make a commitment to running is that they don't realize that their bodies probably haven't been used in years.

Walking helps the body make the transition to the greater stress of running. Although the amount of walking required varies greatly, a couple of weeks of walking only and then a running-walking program is usually the best approach.

Whatever reason you have for walking, here are some tips to get you going in the right direction.

Wear the right shoes. Sneakers are the usual walking shoes, but enlightened shoe companies now market attractive casual and even dress shoes made for walking.

Unburden yourself. Keep your arms free by carrying your belongings in a backpack.

Take advantage of down time. I find that the more I sit, the more tired I get. I spend a lot of time in airports, and I've walked in most of them. It's good for the circulation, to pass the time, and to people-watch. And it beats drinking coffee and eating muffins. The Atlanta airport is excellent for walking. I have calculated that it is 1 mile from one end of the concourses to the other—and it's all carpeted. The Pittsburgh airport is good, too. To accommodate your walking, invest in luggage with wheels.

Shun automatic transportation. Some airports have subways or moving walkways. Similarly, many malls and other large buildings have escalators or elevators. I prefer to get where I'm going on my own two feet, and walking there doesn't take much longer than riding.

Walk throughout the day. If you are busy, figure out ways to get in extra exercise by walking. Combine errands, pick up or drop off the kids at school (you can racewalk or jog home), or schedule your work appointments with an extra 15 minutes built in so that you can walk to your destination if possible.

Spend a family weekend (or vacation) on a walk or hike. The terrain is usually tougher on hikes, and you'll carry extra weight if you wear a pack. A common and popular Norwegian vacation consists of walking in the countryside from one cottage to another. I used to spend hours hiking with my brothers and niece and nephews. As you become fitter, you will enjoy the sights and conversation as you walk.

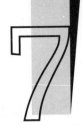

Serious Training
Take It to the Next Level

Have you reached a point in your running where you find yourself motivated beyond doing the minimum? Do you find yourself determined to hit the road despite adverse weather conditions or other impediments? Do you participate in races or want to try? Do you feel that the effort you put into your training doesn't give you the results you want?

If you answered these questions in the affirmative, you are, or want to be, more serious about your running. The definition of *serious* in this case has nothing to do with ability or fast times; it has to do with motivation. If you are running more than my basic program, or you want to, then you are running for reasons beyond health. Perhaps you want to work on getting fitter or to complete a certain race distance or run a certain race time. If so, this chapter is for you.

What spurs a person to get more serious is highly individual, but I have found that no matter what a person's level of ability, motivation must come from within, or it will not last. Whether you're a 4-hour marathoner or an elite competitor, your success in taking your running to the next level is highly dependent on how motivated you are.

Building Up

If you are new to what I call fitness running, allow yourself at least six weeks to build a running base. As you increase your intensity or length of running, remember this important rule: Increase your training by no more than 10 percent per week. Also, make sure you follow the hard day/easy day principle. Following each day of intense effort, take a day off or use "active rest" by cross-training (swimming, walking, or doing some other nonrunning activity).

If you are healthy and basically fit with a running base, you can try speedwork—running faster than a comfortable pace. Speedwork makes you a more efficient runner by allowing you to perform longer at a faster pace. It also adds variety to your training. When to add speedwork to your program is an individual decision based on age and previous fitness, but I would say that, minimally, when you are able to run 4 miles consistently without problems, you can try it. I prescribe a heart rate monitor when you're using speedwork. If you decide to use speedwork to achieve a goal, give it at least six weeks to be effective.

As a cornerstone of faster running, speedwork comes in many forms. Here are some terms and styles of this type of training.

Interval training. This is running with periodic switching between exertion and rest or between a high workload and a low workload. Intervals are a structured system of speedwork usually done on a track or other measured area and at 85 to 90 percent of maximum heart rate (MHR). Intervals are measurable, and thus they tell you more about your fitness level. It is also easier to measure your improvement with intervals. For example, let's say you run 10 quarter miles at 80 seconds per quarter and 85 to 90 percent MHR, with 1 minute of recovery between quarters. Two weeks later, if you do the same workout with the same MHR but your time is 76 seconds per quarter mile, you'll know that with the same physical effort, you are going faster.

Fartlek. Swedish for "speed play," fartlek is a less structured version of interval training, but it is based on the same principles. Fartlek consists of segments of exertion and rest for random distances or times, and it is done off the track. You speed up and slow down as you feel like it. As a hard workout, it can be done at 85 to 90 percent of MHR. Fartlek is less exact than interval training; it can be done in a million different ways. It helps your mind and body adapt to any change of pace that may occur in a race.

Sustained running. This is done over longer distances (2 miles and up) at about 80 to 85 percent of MHR. It is usually run 15 to 30 seconds per mile faster than your comfortable pace.

The Chase Corporate Challenge Program

The following running program was created for the thousands of runners in the Chase Corporate Challenge, an event for which I serve as spokesperson. It includes a series of 3.5-mile races from May to October in 17 cities and 3 countries. Employees of any corporation may participate. Runners are self-scored, and prizes are awarded to individuals and coed and single-sex company teams. The Chase Corporate Challenge training program was specifically designed at the request of the participating runners to help them run faster. These runners vary in age from 30 to 50 and run about 25 miles per week. Ninety percent of them run three to five days a week. In this program, there is no difference in training for men and women.

Over the years, I have observed a lot of the Chase Corporate Challenge races. Many of the male runners finish in the range of 20 to 22 minutes (a pace of about 7 minutes per mile). Many of the women finish at about 25 minutes (8 minutes per mile). These people run regularly but may not be getting the maximum benefit for the time they spend training. After talking to the runners, I realized that almost all of their training is done at the same pace. They have very little variety in their training programs. In other words, they have not tried speed training.

A distance of 3.5 miles is ideal for people with limited time to train. Running a good race at this distance requires a mixture of speed and endurance. To run faster over 3.5 miles, participants have to do some speed training once or twice a week. Running about 25 miles a week, with one to two speed sessions per week, makes a person quite competitive in the Chase Corporate Challenge.

Use my training program as a guideline, then make your own adjustments as necessary. All training should be flexible and adapted to your needs. Be prepared to adjust your program based on weather conditions, available facilities, your health, your job, and family obligations. But don't be overly accommodating so that you lose consistency and discipline.

In the program, the *building phase* is the four- to eight-week period before a race. The *sharpening phase* is during the racing season, or within two to three weeks of the race. If you do not have time for a 5-K race, run a time trial as a gauge. Pick a 5-K or 3-mile route and time yourself running it at your best effort.

The four days are separated by rest, cross-training, or easy running. Any hard running should always be preceded by a substantial warm-up and cool-down period.

Day 1. Five- to 6-mile run at a comfortable pace (75 percent of MHR).

Day 2. Interval training or speedwork. Alternate among the three workouts listed below. They all achieve the same purpose, but variety is important. If you always train in hilly areas, it is okay to skip the hill workout. If you don't run on hills, do the hill workout at least every other week.

- Six to 8 x 400 meters at a 5-K race pace with a 40- to 60-second recovery in the building phase (at or near 85 percent of MHR). Faster than a 5-K pace with a 1½- to 2-minute recovery in the sharpening phase (at or near 90 percent of MHR).
- Four to 6 x 800 meters at a 5-K race pace with a 1½-minute recovery in the building phase. Faster than a 5-K pace with a 2- to 2½-minute recovery in the sharpening phase. Maximum heart rates are the same as the first workout.
- Hill workout: 10 to 12 x 200 meters (85 to 90 percent of MHR, depending on the steepness and length of the hill). Jog back down as a recovery.

Day 3. Seven- to 8-mile run at a comfortable pace (75 percent of MHR).

Day 4. Five miles total, with six to eight pickups that last from 30 seconds to 2½ minutes. Listen to your body and run according to how you feel. This workout is not intended to be as hard as Day 2's. On subsequent fourth days, you can do the following workout. Run 2 miles at a comfortable pace, followed by 2 miles fast (85 percent of MHR). Finish with 1 to 2 miles at a comfortable pace (75 percent of MHR).

Tips from the Top

A time trial can help you assess your conditioning. It also can give you confidence. In 1975, I didn't believe my husband, Jack, when he told me that I could break the world record in only my second 3000-meter race. To convince myself that I had a chance, he had me run a 2000-meter time trial. When I realized that I had only to keep up that trial pace for another 1000 meters and that I could even slow down a little to set the record, I was convinced. I broke the record once that year and again in 1976. Keep in mind that you normally run a bit faster in a race than in a time trial.

With the above program in mind, here are some suggestions to ensure that you train effectively and safely.

Prepare for speed. Do a warm-up and careful stretching before beginning the speed section of your workout.

Use visualization. To be mentally prepared, it helps to go through your speedwork in your mind before doing it.

Choose your training site. Speedwork can be just as convenient as regular running. You can do speedwork anywhere; you don't need a track. If you know your time for a quarter mile or other distance, run that time and mark off the section of road you cover for repeats. You can measure longer distances with your car.

Make sure to rest after a hard day. In addition, don't plan a tough workout on a stressful day, such as a taxing workday or when other major obligations are scheduled.

Work out wisely. On your rest days, whether you choose to cross-train or not to exercise at all should depend on your time and energy. Particularly if you are new to this type of training or have a busy schedule, you must constantly be aware of the danger of overdoing it.

Keeping Track

To construct and analyze your program successfully, keep track of what you do. For the entire 20 years of my competitive career, I kept a diary of my running. I still have these diaries, dating all the way back to 1970.

Keeping a diary is helpful for all levels of runners. Beginners—the most rapidly and consistently improving group—can gain motivation and inspiration by noting their progress. For the more advanced, the diary serves as an instructive and guiding tool for future training. Even for those with significant running experience, a diary is useful. Over time, we almost always forget exactly what we have done. Reviewing past experience helps lead us to where we want to go.

I used my running diary as a tool. Keeping and consulting my diary helped make me a successful runner. The most common training mistake I made during my career was running too hard. Sometimes this was obvious during my workout (if I started my intervals too fast, I couldn't complete them all in the same time or I had to extend the recovery time). At other times, the effect was more subtle, or cumulative, over a longer period. If I experienced problems in training or racing, I could look back over my diaries and find out why by tracing a pattern or spotting a mistake (a day I didn't rest, for example). Conversely, when I was running very well, I could look back to find out what had led to my success in the hope of repeating it.

I think a diary is useful for speed training and racing, but with time and experience, you need not be as exact in recording your easier, or recovery, days. Some runners feel the need to keep a precise account of all of their training. Liz McColgan, an elite marathoner whom I coach, can report to me every detail of her easy runs. I always tell her that I don't need the technical details, just how she feels. I've noticed other runners who click their stopwatches off for the 15 seconds or so that they stop at a red light. While I kept careful track of quality training, I was never quite that exact. Today I time myself in much the same way I did for my easier days in the past: I glance at the clock when I leave the house for a run and check it again when I return. Rather than recording exact times for every run, writing down how you feel in relation to your training might be more useful.

The table on page 80 contains a two-week account of my training during the fourth and third weeks before the 1988 New York City Marathon, which I won in 2:28:06. I include this sample to show how I recorded my training and interspersed hard and easy efforts. As you see, I trained hard on Tuesdays and Saturdays, put forth a medium effort on Thursdays, and had recovery days in between. Again, keep in mind that *recovery* is a relative term; for a world-class runner, it still represents significant mileage.

Reasons to Race

What motivates a person to race? In the beginning, it is a new adventure. The fanfare and camaraderie surrounding a typical road race is a great experience. It is a way to celebrate your fitness and to enjoy the trappings of competition: getting an official time and perhaps a certificate, medal, or T-shirt. And if you keep at it, it is satisfying to experience your improvement, which is usually fairly consistent.

What brings back the veteran road racer, someone who has done it for a while and whose progress may have leveled off? Only a few runners can win their age-group categories, so something else must be bringing out the masses. In addition to the camaraderie and fun, racing often helps people maintain the motivation to train. I also think it gives the average person a chance to feel like an athlete.

Consider one associate of mine, a man who used to weigh 250 pounds. Some years after taking up running, he is slim and fairly fast—and quite addicted to road races. I think the races are his security against slipping back into his former life. I've met other people in their fifties who I've assumed are lifelong athletes, only to learn that they were formerly very overweight. I think continuing to race helps them to maintain their new identities as athletic people. And those who are former athletes can hold on to their old identities by continuing to compete.

Grete's Diary

Mon. 10/10:	A.M.: **8 miles, easy**	
	P.M.: **7 miles and strides, easy**	
Tues. 10/11:	A.M.: **7 miles, easy**	
	P.M.: **2½ miles, 12 x 500 meters, recovery 40 sec.**	
	3 miles	*on the road*
Wed. 10/12:	**14 miles**	*felt heavy-legged*
Thurs. 10/13:	A.M.: **8 miles**	
	P.M.: **2½ miles, 3 x 2000 meters (in 6:20), recovery 2½ min.**	
	2 miles	*on treadmill because of bad weather; felt okay*
Fri. 10/14:	A.M.: **6 miles**	
	P.M.: **7 miles and strides**	
Sat. 10/15:	**2½-mile warm-up, 10-K cross-country race (32:45), 4-mile cool-down**	*very happy with time considering a heavy training week*
Sun. 10/16:	**21 miles**	
Total:	**108 to 110 miles**	
Mon. 10/17:	A.M.: **8 miles**	
	P.M.: **7 miles and strides**	
Tues. 10/18:	**Like Tuesday 10/11**	
Wed. 10/19:	**14 miles**	
Thurs. 10/20:	**10 miles**	
Fri. 10/21:	A.M.: **7 miles**	
	P.M.: **2½-mile warm-up, 3 x 3000 meters, recovery 3 min., 2½-mile cool-down**	*on the road; tough workout*
Sat. 10/22:	A.M.: **8 miles**	
	P.M.: **7 miles and strides**	
Sun. 10/23:	**20 miles**	*felt good all week*
Total:	**105 to 108 miles**	

The following week, I tapered to 87 miles. The week before the marathon, I ran substantially less than that.

Women especially gain greatly by running in road races because so few of them have had the opportunity to be athletes. I often meet women who have made great gains through running and racing. Many surprise themselves. When they start, they don't think of themselves as competitive (nor have they been socialized to be; often the opposite is true). As they get fitter, they become more competitive, first with themselves, then perhaps with others. Every year, a friend's wife competes in the Grete Waitz Run. She started running with the other housewives in her area, and her ambitions grew with her fitness. Now this mother of two, who never had an opportunity to compete in sports before, runs my 5-K race in 21 to 22 minutes, an excellent time.

Tips from the Top

In Norway, we have a very descriptive expression for keeping your cool: "You need to have a bucket of ice cubes in your stomach." To help you do this, remember these tips:

Keep your mind in the present. It's okay to let your thoughts drift in random training (I did) but not in serious training or during a race.

Focus on putting all your energy into running forward. I know this sounds strange, but there are always distractions.

Talk to yourself. I did this constantly, telling myself to stay relaxed and to keep focused. Some people tell themselves to "stay tough" or "relax and focus." Use whatever "conversation" feels right to you.

Look at the runner in front of you. Focus on the person's back, not his shoes, to make sure you are looking forward, which is a more positive and less distracting direction than looking down or away.

There are many reasons to continue racing. Although you can't always get faster, you can find new motivation. My brother Jan keeps running marathons at age 53, mostly because he loves to travel and do them abroad. He knows that he will never be as fast as he once was and that he would not be motivated to train for events in Oslo. But as long as he thinks about running in New York City or Honolulu, he will keep at it.

Racing also comes with other benefits. Often people who race join running clubs, which provide them with both social and running support. I know more than a few avid runners whose families don't share their running joys and aspirations, but in a club, they find others who do. The Chase Corporate Challenge has shown that working toward a race with a group also creates a supportive and bonding atmosphere in the workplace.

Age-Group Competition

When I turned 40, people constantly asked if I would compete as a masters runner. People actually started asking this question a few years before I reached this "magic age." That type of competition never interested me, mostly because I knew I could never run faster than I had in my prime. By the time I retired from competition, I felt satisfied with what I had done. Although it was difficult at first to imagine myself not doing the thing I knew best, I eventually felt ready to let go of the life I had led.

Often successful masters runners are those who were not previously competitive. Their bodies and their motivation are fresher. Some formerly elite runners start out "hot" in the masters category, but they don't stay at the top for long. The only exception I can think of, over the long term at least, is Bill Rodgers, who has made a successful career of both open and masters running.

For those who keep running, especially into the older age-groups, placing well in their group or winning an age award is a great goal. And when and if they do, it is a satisfying and exciting outcome of their efforts.

The Marathon

The marathon was the centerpiece of my "second career" (after track running). Why did I decide to run it? The first time, in 1978, I was offered a ticket to New York City. As a top track runner, the organizers thought I'd make a good "rabbit" (pacesetter) for the favorites. Since I had never run longer than 12 miles, I guess they figured that was about as far as I could go, but at least I'd do it quickly. I accepted the offer because I had never been to the United States and Jack and I wanted to see the sights. Later in my career, success kept me going the distance. I didn't race to earn a living at first, as that possibility didn't really exist. For the first three years of my marathoning career, I also taught school full-time.

Some of my reasons for running the marathon are the same as those of other runners. The distance is a challenge. Doing it well is a challenge. Winning it is an even bigger challenge. After running on the track, the marathon was new territory. I knew my track career had limits, and I wanted to see where this new avenue would

Are You Ready to Run a Marathon?

Even if your motivation to run a marathon is sound, you need to be in the proper physical condition. I think you should be running for at least one year before attempting a marathon. A lot of programs and experts say that you can do it with less training, but that depends on your fitness level. If you have a fitness base, are in your twenties, or have a large amount of time to invest in training, perhaps it is possible to run a marathon in less than a year. But if you're starting from scratch, at least a year of training is a safe bet. Besides, after that time, you'll be in great shape. You will have integrated running into your life, you'll have an idea of the commitment it takes to run 26.2 miles, and your body will know how to respond to the major stress of a marathon.

take me. And although I swore to Jack "never again" after crossing the finish line of my first marathon, I was especially motivated by breaking a world record on my first try. I broke the world record three more times, but my primary goal wasn't breaking records; my goal was winning. As time went on, the competition became very stiff, and my most difficult victories motivated me even more.

For many people, the marathon is a mystery. The thought of running 26.2 miles is daunting, and just finishing is the goal. In addition, training requires a lot of time and energy. And unlike races at shorter distances, if you don't succeed, you can't do another one a week later. I try to emphasize this in clinics and to encourage people to set aside a lot of time to get ready. I realize that since millions of people have run at least one marathon, newcomers may be more casual about attempting one. Those are often the people who struggle across the finish line after 5 or 6 hours. I think most people can get much more satisfaction from doing their homework and being properly prepared to run the race.

I ran 16 marathons over the course of my career—not that many when you stop to think about it. I usually ran only one a year, a few times two. Serious runners rarely, if ever, do more than two per year. The marathon is a very strenuous physical and mental test. For some people, once is enough. A 50-year-old former 400-meter runner I know wanted to try a marathon for years. Finally, he entered the New York City Marathon. He did everything right: He prepared properly and ran the first half of the race conservatively, holding back. He completed the distance in 4 hours and was very satisfied with his effort. When I asked him whether he wanted to do another one, he said that he was very happy with experiencing it just once.

I've been asked if I got more satisfaction from winning a marathon than from winning other races. I was very happy to win a 3000-meter race. Winning is always satisfying. But when you succeed in a marathon, it's a bigger victory. The physical reminders of running that distance stay with you for a while, and the feeling of achievement is sweeter and lasts longer because you've put so much effort into it.

Successful Racing

People who run almost every day and use different training techniques with the intention of competing are racers. They also may run for fitness and fun, but their chief goals are to do well in races and to improve their times.

Successful racing is a combination of many factors. I wish I could bottle a formula for feeling great the whole way and having everything under control. To be able to do your best in a race, you must peak for it, which means preparing yourself to be at your fittest and freshest for the race. To do that, you have to cut back on training as the race approaches (this is called *tapering*), sharpen your speed, and get sufficient rest.

Tapering plays a key role in racing success. I used to cut back to one easy run per day several days before an important event and do even less the day before it. Rest or easy training makes your body hungrier to race, and it is much more exciting to race when you're rested and ready to go. Many runners are afraid of resting; sometimes it takes just as much discipline to rest as it does to run. If I could go back and do one thing differently in my career, I would rest more.

Tips from the Top

Being focused was very important in my racing. I learned this when I was running on the track. A track race is so fast and so intense that you can't afford to lose your concentration for even a second. Concentration plays an important role in road racing as well, as so many things can distract you. Remember to stay relaxed and to concentrate on the next mile marker or landmark. During the race, I used to tell myself to stay calm and focused and to run relaxed. Practice this focus in training.

Pacing is an important part of successful running. The type of pacing you use in a race depends on personal preference and experience. Some runners prefer going out fast and hanging on to the end, while others have greater success with even pacing. The experts say that even-paced racing is the most physiologically efficient.

My experience in going out fast in races was usually disastrous. Running at an even pace was more successful for me. I like to be in control throughout a race. You lose this control when you go out too fast and must struggle to the finish.

Having a great race keeps all of us running. Success depends on a number of factors. Some things we can't control, such as weather, the course, and the competition. But some things we can control. Here are some tips on the things you can control in a race. If you follow these tips, your races will be enjoyable and memorable.

Make a plan and stick to it. You should plan everything from how you'll get to the race site to how you'll run the race. When you pack your racing gear, make sure that you have everything you'll need and that it's tried-and-true. Don't be tempted to try new shoes or a new prerace diet; these things should be tested in training. Stick to what you know works for you.

Be mentally prepared. This is essential to running a great race. Picture the upcoming race course, your competition, and your goal. Create a mental image of yourself as a powerful runner.

Pack a snack in your bag. Sometimes a snack won't be available after the race. Having something to eat after your effort will speed your recovery.

Arrive early. Give yourself time to sign up, warm up, find the baggage check, and go to the bathroom. If you are afraid that water will not be available at the start, bring your own.

Warm up. The shorter the race, the longer you'll need to warm up. I used to warm up (light jogging and stretching) for about 30 minutes before a 5-K race and 15 minutes for a longer run, such as a marathon.

Do your full stretching routine. This is especially critical for shorter distances because the pace is quicker and you'll need greater flexibility to achieve your full range of motion and prevent injury.

Position yourself correctly at the starting line. Don't stand in the front row if you don't belong there. Doing so is unfair to faster racers and may cause you to go out too quickly. Likewise, don't position yourself among slower runners.

Don't be a rabbit. Starting out too fast and going into oxygen debt very quickly will short-circuit your race plans. Racing requires constant concentration, particularly at shorter distances. In longer races, you have more time to distribute your energy equally. The challenge is often keeping focused and not succumbing to fatigue in the middle stretch.

Cool down. After a race, the last thing you may feel like doing is more running. But just as in training, you need to at least walk off the fatigue from your effort.

Change your clothes. To prevent a chill and possible illness and to keep your muscles warm, put on dry clothes as soon as possible after the race.

Be respectful of your running. A race is often an effort beyond even hard training. Allow yourself plenty of rest and recovery, perhaps more than what you are accustomed to.

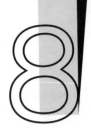

Stretching
and Strengthening
Achieving Exercise Balance

This chapter was written with the assistance of Gerard Hartmann, my massage and sports injury therapist. Gerard, formerly of Gainesville, Florida, is now living back in his native Ireland. He has a master's degree in science and kinesiotherapy and treats many world-class athletes. Gerard also is an accomplished athlete—a seven-time Irish national triathlon champion.

In previous chapters, I dealt with the cardiovascular aspects of exercise. But there is another element to the fitness equation. The key to healthy, overall fitness is the balance created by muscle flexibility and strength. This can be ensured by adding the exercises I describe in this chapter to your program.

The Need to Stretch

I admit that I have not always been conscientious enough about stretching. I'm afraid this is the case with more than a few world-class runners. Although I probably should have stretched more in my competitive days, I can't dispute the importance of doing so. Stretching has numerous benefits for overall fitness.

- ↳ It lessens the risk of injury by increasing the range of motion.
- ↳ It reduces muscle soreness by improving circulation and the flushing out of metabolic wastes.
- ↳ It increases flexibility, which is especially important as we age and our muscles become less elastic.

My husband, Jack, has enlightened me on the need to stretch, but not in a way you might expect. He has never stretched, and even now, when he tries to bend over to stretch the back of his thighs, he is so tight that his body remains at a 90-degree angle. Over the years, Jack has hurt his back and has had a sore knee, a sore Achilles tendon, and a number of other aches and pains. He has usually solved these problems by taking a few days off from running. Finally, when Jack was 49, Gerard Hartmann prescribed a stretching program for him. Although he's a bit more flexible now, for the most part, you can't teach that old dog new tricks.

I have found that women are generally more disciplined about stretching than men. I'm not sure why this is so. Perhaps it is easier for them to stretch because they are inherently more flexible. Or perhaps many took dance or gymnastics lessons as young girls or did other activities where stretching and flexibility were emphasized.

Running takes a big toll on flexibility, since the movement is restrictive and repetitive. Running also is very hard on the body because of the constant pounding. That's why it is so important to stretch and strengthen certain muscles if you are a runner. But stretching should be included in any exercise program, no matter what the activity. And for beginners, it's especially beneficial to develop good habits from the start.

I have to admit that I still do not spend enough time stretching and strengthening. Sometimes I get out of my routine or get lazy. Then I dread starting up again because I know I'll be sore. In recent years, as I have become better educated on this subject and have learned that flexibility decreases with age, I have devoted more time to these exercises.

The exercises I prescribe here are not a burden for the busy exerciser. They should take only about 10 minutes and can be done practically anywhere. If you are pressed for time, it is better to cut your workout a bit short than to cut down on stretching and strengthening.

My current system of stretching is called *active-isolated stretching*. It entails isolating the muscles and stretching them for a short period of time (3 to 8 seconds). This form of stretching has three main steps. First, the body is put in the safest anatomical position. This is essential, since more harm than good is done by stretching incorrectly. Second, the muscle to be stretched is isolated with precise localized movements, thus enhancing flexibility. Third, holding the stretch for shorter periods and doing repetitions of the same stretch increase blood and oxygen flow to the tissues being stretched. This encourages the muscle to lengthen and provides more flexibility than if you held the stretch longer. In a longer stretch, the muscle becomes fatigued and, in a protective fashion, fights the stretch.

At what point in your workout should you stretch? For many years, the prevailing theory was that you should stretch only when the muscles were warmed up (after at least 10 minutes of exercise) or right after a workout. Stretching after exercising allows you to regain flexibility after doing your main activity's limited range of motion. Recent studies indicate that stretching itself can also be a warm-up. As long as you don't use bouncing, jerky movements or stretch too quickly, you can safely stretch for 5 to 10 minutes before exercising.

I like to stretch after a post-exercise cool-down and shower. After an intense workout, my muscles are tired and may go into spasm if I stretch too soon.

Active-Isolated Stretches

Following are six simple stretches that will ensure flexible muscles and reduce your chances of injury. Unless otherwise indicated, hold all stretches for 5 to 8 seconds and repeat each exercise five to eight times. Always stretch until you feel a slight irritation. Never stretch to the point of pain.

Hamstring Stretches

In 1991, I began to have some problems with my back thigh muscles. My lack of care for these muscles during my competitive career probably aggravated the situation. It began with pain, which I tried to ignore, in the area where the hamstring meets the pelvis. Then the pain became chronic, and it got to the point where I couldn't run at all. Inflexible and weak hamstring muscles were the cause.

Gerard had to break up the scar tissue in the area with deep friction massage. Then he prescribed a stretching and strengthening routine done with cuff weights. This is the hamstring stretch he prescribed. You will need a short length of rope or a towel for this stretch.

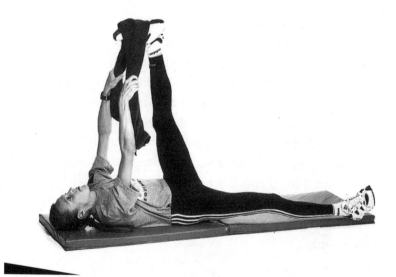

Lie on your back with your legs straight. Lift your left leg, keep it straight, and use the strength of your quadriceps (front thigh muscle) to pull your leg up as far as you can. When you can extend the leg no farther, take the rope or towel and drape it over the bottom of your left foot. Hold the two ends of the rope or towel and gently pull your left leg toward your head until you feel the stretch. Concentrate on relaxing the hamstring muscle. Release to the nonstretch position while keeping the left leg straight. Switch legs and repeat.

Muscles stretch to the best advantage when they are relaxed. Many people stretch the hamstrings by standing up, propping the leg on a chair or table, and then leaning over. If you stretch the hamstring in a stand-up position (as opposed to lying down), you will not achieve the maximum flexibility because the muscle is contracting. Sitting to do the stretch is not quite as bad as standing, but it is still not the best position.

Gluteal Muscle Stretches

I did this exercise religiously in my competitive days. I think all runners have a tendency to experience tightness in the buttocks and lower back area. I am particularly aware of the tightness in this area when I get a massage.

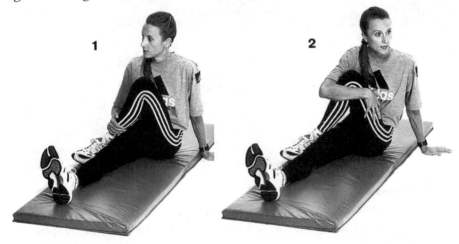

1. Sit on the floor with the right leg extended and the left leg bent. Cross your left foot over the straight leg and place it next to the outside of the right knee.

2. Wrap your right arm around the outside of the left knee. Then twist your trunk to the left and gently pull the knee toward your chest. You should feel the stretch in the buttocks muscle on the left side of the body. Switch legs and repeat.

Quadriceps Stretches

I never had a problem with my front thigh muscles when I was running, but when I started biking a lot, I experienced more tightness there. Gerard showed me this exercise, and I've been much more flexible ever since.

Many people do this exercise by standing on one leg, bending the other knee, and pulling the foot toward the buttocks. When stretching this way, you must either bend forward (lessening the stretch) or arch your lower back. Again, the object is to stretch the muscle in its most relaxed position.

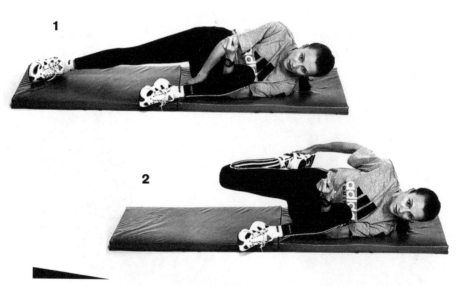

1. Lie on your left side and extend your right leg. Bring your left knee to your chest by hooking your left arm under the knee. This stabilizes the spine and pelvis.

2. With your right hand, pull your right foot toward your buttocks. Switch legs and repeat.

Calf Stretches

I have always done the standard wall stretch for my calves. If a stair is available, I'll sometimes stand on it with the front part of my foot and lower my heel to stretch the calf. In line with his other stretches, Gerard suggests a calf stretch while sitting.

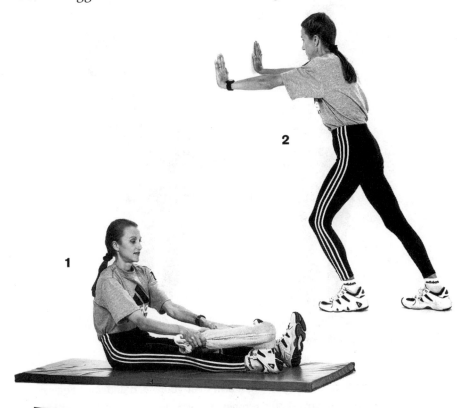

1. Sit on the floor and extend your legs. Drape a rope or towel over your right foot and pull back on the toes until you feel the stretch in your calf. You can bend the left knee if it is more comfortable. Switch legs and repeat.

2. Facing the wall at arm's length, place your right leg 1 to 2 feet behind the other leg. Lean on the wall and keep the right leg straight and the left knee bent. Keeping your right heel on the ground and your back straight, slowly lean into the wall. Switch legs and repeat. To stretch the lower calf and Achilles tendon, do the same stretch, but bend the right knee.

Lateral Trunk Stretches

This is a good upper-body stretch that works the muscles of the upper back, chest, hips, shoulders, and neck.

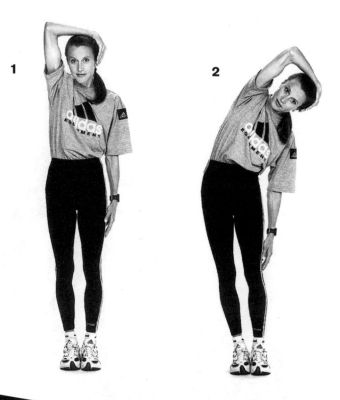

1   2

1. While standing, extend your right arm over your head and lay it against your left ear. Your left arm should remain at your side.

2. Lean to your left until your left arm extends down to the side of your left knee. Switch arms and repeat.

Triceps Stretches

This is often called the "scratch your back" stretch. It creates more flexibility in the muscle at the back of the upper arm.

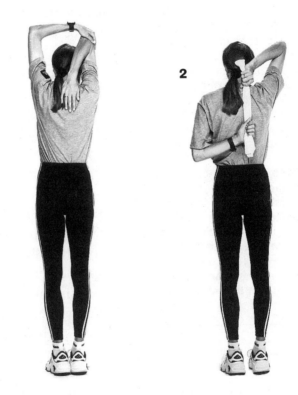

1. While standing, bend your right arm so that you can reach your right hand down your back. Reach over your head with your left hand, grasp your right elbow, and gently push back on the right elbow. Switch arms and repeat.

2. A variation for those who are more limber is to reach for your right hand by bringing your left hand up your back toward the right hand. You can assist this process by dropping a towel down your back and grabbing it with your left hand.

Fast Fitness

People often spend the entire day hunched over in activities such as driving, watching television, talking on the telephone, and doing exercises such as push-ups and swimming. To open up the chest and shoulders, stand in a doorway, grasp the two sides of the frame, and walk out far enough so that your arms are behind you. Hold for 5 seconds and repeat six times. A good time to perform this stretch is after a warm shower or bath, when your body temperature is high.

This is also a good time to relieve tension in the neck and shoulder muscles. Hold your chin to your chest and gently flex your head forward with your hands. Next, use one hand to gently pull your head toward a shoulder. Do the same on the other side. These stretches are physically relaxing, and they'll give you a sense of well-being.

Strengthening Exercises

Concentrating on balanced muscle strengthening, which can be done with resistance exercises, really pays off. As we age, particularly after 35, we experience a slight decrease in muscle mass, strength, aerobic capacity, and metabolism. If you stay active, these attributes will deteriorate much more slowly than if you are sedentary. Strengthening the muscles helps build bone density, which also diminishes with age, and prevents osteoporosis.

Resistance exercise takes some commitment. To get results, strengthening exercises must be done at least twice a week. Doing them once a week won't have much effect. For busy people, I have provided two strengthening options. The first four exercises are a minimal routine, which should be done in tandem with the stretching exercises. The rest are optional additions. Keeping in mind that time is of the essence, if you think you have only enough time to do your aerobic exercise, I recommend cutting this portion back by 10 minutes to accommodate some strengthening exercises.

Most people condition only the muscles they use in their exercise or sport. To illustrate how this can create imbalances, consider a radical example: marathon runners. I say radical because although most of them are extraordinarily fit, the average marathoner lacks upper-body muscle tone. Many professional runners of my era, including me, began strength programs in our mid-thirties, relatively late in our careers.

With minimal effort—doing just the following few exercises—you can guarantee more balanced strength. The basic strengthening routine should be done three to five times a week. Crunches, however, can be done every day if you wish. Also, you should stretch the muscles after strengthening them. Again, crunches are an exception, as the muscles worked are too deep to obtain a stretch.

Crunches

Many exercisers don't understand how important strong abdominal muscles are. These muscles do more than define your stomach area; they also protect your lower back. Ninety percent of us will encounter back pain at some point in our lives, and most of that pain will be from weak muscles.

To appreciate the positive side of having strong, firm abdominals, look at the negative side. For every 10 pounds of weight on the front of the stomach, 10 times that amount of pressure is exerted on the lower back.

A true sit-up—coming up so that your entire back is off the ground—works the hip flexors. But it is the trunk flexors you want to strengthen, and they are worked in only the first 20 percent of a sit-up. You can strengthen the trunk flexors by rising only to the point of feeling the muscle contract, with just the shoulders and upper back coming off the floor. This slighter rise is called a crunch. For abdominal strengthening, limit your exercise to crunches rather than sit-ups. Do two or three sets (with 15 to 20 crunches per set) of each type of crunch per session.

Beware of doing crunches on a slant board. This will work the hip flexors, which are generally five to six times stronger in most people than the trunk flexors.

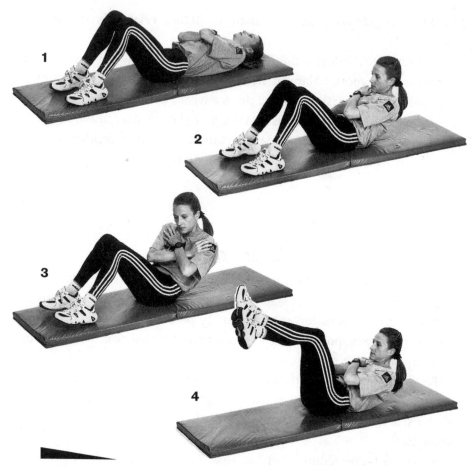

1. Lie on the ground, bend your knees, keep your feet flat on the floor, and cross your hands on your chest. (Clasping your hands behind your head can strain your neck, because people tend to tug on the neck. It's fine to put your hands on the side of your head.)

2. Raise up without twisting until your shoulders and upper back are off the floor. Then slowly lower yourself to the beginning position. Repeat 15 to 20 times.

3. Do another set of 15 to 20 crunches, but work different abdominal muscles by touching the elbow to the opposite thigh.

4. To increase the benefits, I like to add alternating sets of a more complex crunch. Keeping your knees bent, raise your legs in the air and cross your ankles. You also can place a 5- or 10-pound weight on your chest while doing the crunches.

Push-ups

I come from the world of running, where most of us look like kangaroos. The bottom half of the body is strong and well-developed, while the top half often looks small and skinny by comparison. If you have unlimited time, you can go to a gym for a full routine of upper body work. But for the busy exerciser, nothing beats the old-fashioned push-up for a quick and total upper body strengthening exercise.

I vary my repetitions depending on how I feel. By doing several sets of 10 to 20 push-ups per session, you'll derive benefits. Spreading your hands farther apart or placing them closer together will strengthen different muscles.

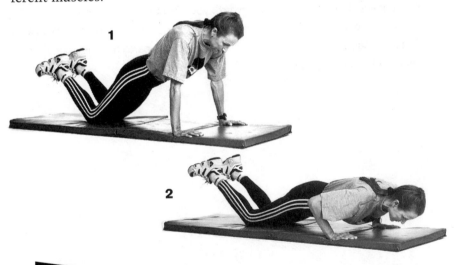

1. Push-ups are difficult. Beginners may want to start by doing them with the knees bent and the feet in the air. I highly recommend putting a mat under your knees to minimize stress on them.

2. Keeping your back straight and your palms flat on the floor, shoulders' width apart, lower yourself until your body is almost parallel to the floor.

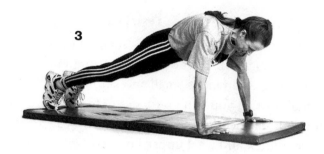

3. Position your body at about a 45-degree angle to the floor, with your weight supported only by your palms and toes. Your palms should be flat on the floor, shoulders' width apart. Keep your elbows slightly bent, not locked. Your fingers should be pointing forward, your feet together. Your legs, back, and neck should be in a straight line, with your face down. Looking up puts a strain on your neck. Lower yourself until your body is parallel to the floor, then return to the starting position.

Lower-Back Strengtheners

My most unfortunate incident of back pain came during the 1984 Olympics in Los Angeles. The two nights before the marathon, I slept in a bed that was very soft. My lower back, which is sometimes problematic, went into spasm. The day before the marathon, I wasn't able to run at all. I spent all day with a doctor and a physical therapist trying to get my back loosened and recovered. By race day, I had gotten over the pain, but the incident prevented me from being 100 percent prepared and focused on the race.

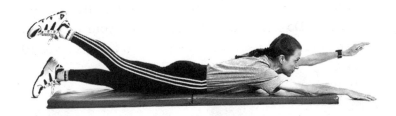

Lie flat on your stomach, legs extended. Lift your right leg about 6 inches off the floor, simultaneously lifting your left arm. Raise your head slightly as you do this. Hold for 2 seconds, then switch to the other leg and arm. Do two or three sets of 10, building up to sets of 20.

Runners and Leg Exercises

If you're a runner, you probably don't need to do leg-strengthening exercises because you work those muscles enough already. However, some runners believe that extra strengthening of the legs is beneficial. If you take this extra step, don't make it a major part of your resistance program. Unless you have an imbalance or a weakness or you are prone to injuries in areas that require strengthened muscles for support (such as the knees), you probably don't need to work your legs. Also, if you run on undulating surfaces (with a good number of hills), you are developing leg strength. Runners are usually stronger in the quadriceps than in other muscles, and that creates an imbalance. I regret that I did not work on strengthening the opposing muscles (the hamstrings) during my career.

Heel Drops

This exercise is a variation of toe raises. Toe raises, which are meant to strengthen the calves, are done by pushing up on your toes. Gerard contends that weak calves are very seldom the cause of injury. He feels that the calf muscle, particularly in runners, is usually sufficiently strong but often not flexible enough. He suggests concentrating on stretching, rather than strengthening, the calves.

Achilles tendinitis, or a calf muscle tear, often results from a weakness in the Achilles tendon, which attaches the calf muscle to the heel bone. Heel drops will solve this problem by strengthening the Achilles tendon. Do this exercise fairly rapidly and rhythmically, and focus on the down portion. Do not raise yourself high on your toes when you come back up, and don't use extra weights. Do three sets of 10. You should experience a slight burning sensation in the calves on the third set.

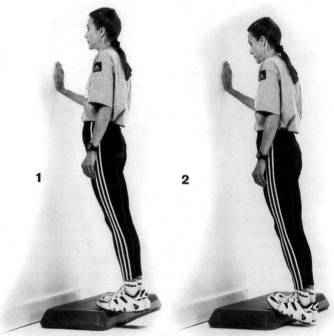

1

2

1. Stand on your toes on a step or similar surface.
2. Let your heels drop down. Rise slightly, then repeat.

Stepping Up Your Strength

No matter what your age or fitness level, you'll be better off with strength training. Routinely doing the stretching and strengthening exercises described in the preceding sections will provide you with all the benefits of having flexible and toned muscles.

But you may want to take your strengthening further. With the additional exercises starting on page 105, you can increase your protection from exercise-induced injuries and universal problems such as lower back, neck, and shoulder pain. Most of these exercises were prescribed for me by Gerard. They not only tone the muscles but aid in good posture. Again, the focus is on fast, easy, efficient, and inexpensive exercise.

If you have access to a club or gym, you can do your weight work there. Health clubs have a variety of fancy weight machines and free weights, but if you don't have the time or money to go to a club, you can do your weight work at home, without buying cumbersome and expensive equipment.

Two 5-pound dumbbells and two 5-pound cuff weights (floppy weights that wrap around your ankles or wrists) are all you need to do the exercises in this chapter. You can find these at your local discount store. The total cost should be no more than $35 to $50.

Do 5 to 15 repetitions of each exercise. If you cannot do 5 repetitions, start the program without weights. You are lifting the right amount and doing the right number of repetitions if you feel muscle fatigue by the third set. As you get stronger, add weight in 5-pound increments and work up to three sets again. After several increments, stay at that amount to maintain strength. The point is to maintain, not

Get Going with Grete

What is aging? It is the loss of strength and an increase in frailty. It also means a gradual loss of muscle mass and a shift in the body's muscle/fat ratio. You can't prevent this process, but you can slow it down by increasing your activity and building your strength. Since muscle weighs more than fat, don't let the scale be your guide after taking up strength training. Judge success by your body shape; just notice how much better your clothes fit.

Fitness Facts

Those who use hand or ankle weights believe that they get a better workout by increasing their workload. But, says Gerard Hartmann, "I don't see the physiological benefit of carrying weights when you run. It changes the natural cadence and form of running or walking. The body was not designed to use weights while doing these activities." Attaching ankle or leg weights also can be dangerous. "It affects the normal running or walking gait, and thus can cause injuries," Gerard adds. He says that moving the arms vigorously during power walking and doing the strengthening exercises in this chapter are better tactics than using weights while exercising.

gain, strength. If you are inspired to increase your strength, Gerard suggests you take up a more serious program at a gym or health club.

For each exercise, lift for 2 to 3 seconds, hold for 1 second, and lower the weight in a 3-second count. Don't make the common mistake of working only the concentric (raising, or toward the body) portion and not the eccentric (lowering, or away from the body) portion by letting gravity do the work.

Outer-Thigh Lifts

This exercise strengthens the muscles of the outer thigh and hip.

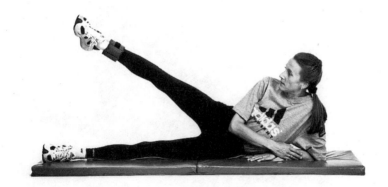

Attach a cuff weight to your right leg. Lie on your left side with both legs extended and prop yourself up on your left arm. Raise your right leg so it is only 45 degrees off the floor, then lower it. Turn over, switch legs and cuff weight, and repeat.

Inner-Thigh Lifts

This exercise strengthens the muscles of the inner thigh and hip.

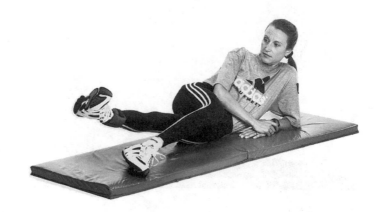

Attach a cuff weight to your left leg. Lie on your left side with both legs extended and prop yourself up on your left arm. Bend your right knee for comfort and rest your right foot on the floor. Lift your left leg, then lower it to the floor. Turn over, switch legs and cuff weight, and repeat.

Hamstring Strengtheners

This exercise is optional for runners, since your thighs are probably strong enough already.

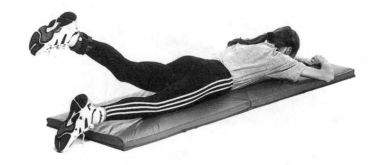

Attach a cuff weight to your left ankle. Lie on your stomach, with your arms extended over your head. Lift your left leg straight up, 8 to 10 inches, depending on how heavy the cuff weight is. Keep your knees straight. Lower your left leg to the floor. Switch legs and cuff weight and repeat.

Quadriceps Strengtheners

Here are two exercises to strengthen the muscles on top of your thigh.

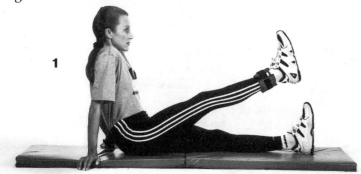

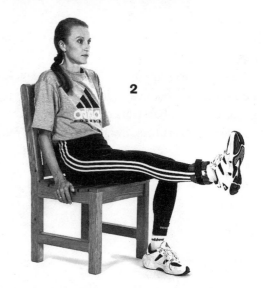

1. Attach a cuff weight to your right ankle. Sit on the floor with your legs extended. Prop yourself up by keeping your hands behind you. Lift your right leg straight up, keeping your knee straight, then lower the leg to the floor. Switch legs and cuff weight and repeat. This works your hip flexors—muscles that let you swing your legs forward and are essential for running.

2. Attach a cuff weight to your right ankle. While sitting in a chair or on a table, lift your right leg until it is straight out, then lower it to the floor. Switch legs and cuff weight and repeat. This works the lower quadriceps.

Shoulder Strengtheners

To develop upper-body strength specific to your sport, why not just hold hand weights while running? Although this is sometimes prescribed, it is not a good idea. Gerard says, "It's too ballistic, too fast, and not controlled." The first activity shown here is a shoulder flexion exercise, which works the biceps and front shoulder muscles.

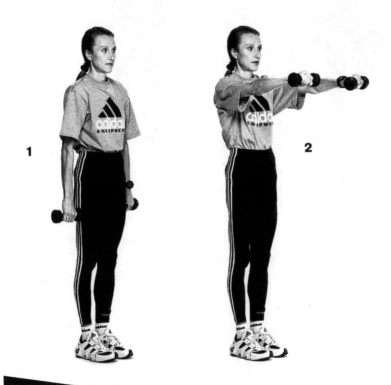

1. Stand straight with a dumbbell in each hand. Hold the dumbbells at your sides, with your palms facing backward.

2. Lift your arms to shoulder height. Lower and repeat.

This exercise works the entire shoulder area.

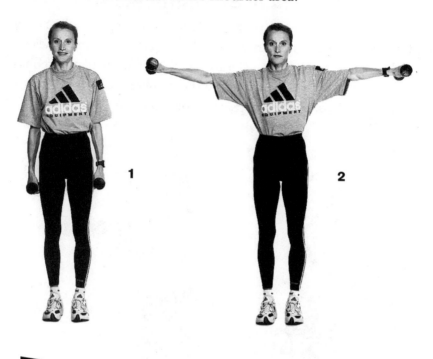

1

2

1. Stand straight with a dumbbell in each hand. Hold the dumbbells at your sides, with your palms facing toward your legs.

2. Lift your arms straight out to the side to shoulder height. Lower and repeat.

Biceps Curls

To strengthen the muscle at the front of the upper arm, this exercise requires movement only at the elbow joint. Do two sets of 20 per arm.

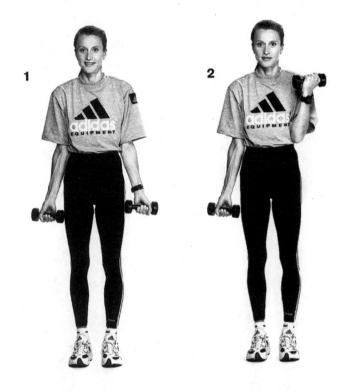

1. Stand straight with a dumbbell in each hand. Hold the dumbbells at your sides, with your palms facing out from your body.

2. Raise your left arm toward your body by bending it at the elbow. Lower, switch arms, and repeat.

Triceps Extensions

This exercise works the muscle at the back of the upper arm. Do both exercises to achieve and maintain balanced strength in your arms. Do two sets of 20 or three sets of 15.

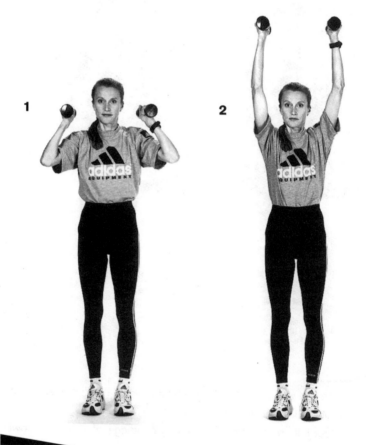

1. Stand straight with a dumbbell in each hand. Hold the dumbbells so that they are next to your ears, palms facing toward your head.

2. Lift the dumbbells over your head until your arms are fully extended. Take care not to arch your lower back. If your weights are heavy, you might want to do this exercise one arm at a time by leaning over a weight bench or chair.

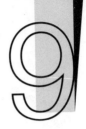

Cross-Training
Variety to Keep You Fresh

When I first became involved in sports as a young girl, my sports club encouraged me to try a variety of activities. In addition to running, I played team handball and went cross-country skiing. I also dabbled in field events, such as the high jump, long jump, hurdles, and—believe it or not—shot put. In my twenties, I competed in some cross-country ski races over 20 to 25 miles, in which I did quite well. During Oslo winters, I often skied instead of running. From my early cross-training activities, I gained a type of true physical education—learning various skills and developing an overall conditioning that I believe greatly contributed to my success as a world-class athlete. This early experience has served me to this day. And what's more, I had a lot of fun.

After focusing on my running for 20 years, it was a pleasure to take up cross-training again. I still consider the multisport lifestyle fun, and I look forward to the change of pace that nonrunning activities provide. I enjoy long hikes with my family and mountain biking with my husband. And these days, I even take advantage of new sports such as deep-water running and in-line skating.

My Cross-Training Week

Following is a sample of my current exercise program, which relies heavily on the multisport approach. In the winter, I tend to run four days rather than five. If I am in Oslo and the weather is bad, I run on a treadmill. In the summer, when the pool water is warm, I may do deep-water running on my days off from road running. Three times a week I use cuff weights to do hamstring-strengthening exercises, push-ups, and crunches. Some weeks I may exercise only three or four days. This example represents a perfect week: no travel, few obligations, and nice weather.

Day 1: Run 6 to 9 miles at a comfortable pace.

Day 2: Same as Day 1.

Day 3: Ride stationary bike for 45 to 60 minutes. If the weather is nice and I have the time, take a 4- to 5-mile walk in the afternoon.

Day 4: Same as Day 1.

Day 5: Ride stationary bike or use cross-country ski machine for 45 to 60 minutes. Afternoon same as Day 3.

Day 6: Same as Day 1.

Day 7: Same as Day 1 or Day 5.

Why It Pays to Cross-Train

What is cross-training, and why do it? Quite simply, cross-training is a combination of two or more sports or types of exercise. It became widely popular with the advent of the triathlon, an endurance event that features swimming, bicycling, and running.

The reasons to cross-train are many: to add variety to a workout; to develop overall, balanced fitness; to prevent injury; and to discover which exercises you like best. Cross-training also is great for weight loss, allowing you to do more exercise without overstressing parts of the body in any single activity. And by resting the muscles from your primary exercise, cross-training allows your body to recover from activity better.

One of the reasons I cross-train is to relieve the stress on my body that comes from all my years of running. When I get carried away, I run every day for a month, up to 50 or 60 miles a week. Then, sure enough, I feel soreness in my knees or tightness in my hamstrings. When I'm cross-training, I keep my running to five days and about 40 miles in a good week. By taking off from running and doing some exercises that focus on the upper body, I create balance and minimize my overall risk of developing soreness or injury from overuse. For these reasons, both my beginning and advanced training programs (see chapters 4 and 7) provide for a couple of days per week of alternative training.

Another benefit of cross-training is that it's very flexible. The last thing those of us with busy lifestyles need is more structure. A nice aspect of my current exercise program is that I train more or less according to how I feel. I enjoy the freedom of picking and choosing among exercise activities, depending on my schedule, the weather, and my mood. This relaxed approach works well for me. I don't feel guilty skipping a day or two of exercise when I'm feeling too tired or busy.

If you're a runner, remember that cross-training can help you to run better, faster, and longer and to run for the rest of your life. I love running, and I want to be able to enjoy it 15 years from now. But if I ran as much as I want to, my body couldn't stand it over the long term. I'm 43, and I've been running for 31 years. Twenty-four of those years included extremely hard running. I put my body through a lot. Even though I like to think of myself as a superwoman, I am at the mercy of my muscles, bones, and joints, just like everyone else.

In terms of wear and tear on the body of a runner, I am in uncharted territory. I believe that I was the first woman runner to train at more than 100 miles a week for the length of my 20-year career. Some men had done it, but for the most part, when they retired, they truly retired. They did not continue any regular form of exercise. I'm surprised when I meet former distance runners who are now completely out of shape. I can't imagine that. I loved the running I did in the past, and I love it just as much now. But I wouldn't be able to do it as much without cross-training.

Training for All Levels

The common lament of beginners is that they become bored with a single exercise, then quit. By taking advantage of the variety of exercises available through cross-training, your chances of sticking with it are better. I advise beginners not to get caught up in specific workouts once they try new activities, get an exercise machine, or join a health club. Start by getting to know the equipment so that you feel comfortable with it. And let yourself play. When I first got my treadmill, I considered it my new toy.

Intermediate athletes benefit from cross-training in the same way as beginners. For example, you can increase your aerobic capacity even while resting your legs from running. Then, when you actually do a running workout, the quality of your running will improve because you are more efficient aerobically. For intermediate athletes, I recommend cross-training at least once a week. If your aim is to increase your fitness, however, you should be proficient enough at the alternative sport to get a good workout from it. For instance, I'm not a good swimmer. Since I can do only the breaststroke, I can't get my heart rate up in the water. That's why I rely on deep-water running, which allows me to copy the workouts I do on the road, except the recovery time after a strenuous effort in the water is shorter than on the road.

In my experience, serious runners are the hardest group to talk into cross-training. Very often, they won't try cross-training until they are injured. If you are a serious runner, realize that you don't really need extra, easy runs. They are usually just junk mileage (easy miles that add volume to your training but don't increase your fitness). You could get the same benefit—if not more—by doing another activity. To save your legs, consider deep-water running or a cross-country ski machine. I intersperse running with two or three of these other workouts each week.

Crossing Over

If you're going to cross over to cross-training, here are some recommended sports and exercise activities to get you started. I do most of these activities. Some are tried-and-true cross-training methods devised by good friends of mine who need workouts that are convenient and time-efficient. Many of the exercises are for the intermediate to serious exerciser, although beginners can work their way up to them. As with running, don't forget to warm up, cool down, and stretch after these activities. And remember that even if you are physically fit from other activities, any new one stresses different muscles and joints, so allow yourself time to get used to a new exercise.

Deep-water running. For this activity, duplicate the running training you do on the road. You just have to de-

---

Get Going with Grete

Try a cycling workout based on fartlek (Swedish for "speed play"). Warm up with a 10-minute easy ride, then play with the levels of the bike to increase the difficulty of the pedaling. (Don't make it too difficult. I make sure I can keep pedaling at 85 rpm.) Do this for 4 minutes. Ease back to a recovery level for 2 to 3 minutes. Then pick a level between the previous two and do a medium ride for 7 to 8 minutes. Then do 5 minutes easy, 5 minutes hard, 2 to 3 minutes easy, and 5 minutes hard. Finish with an easy cool-down for 10 minutes. The total workout is 45 minutes.

---

velop a feel for running in water. Concentrate on simulating the type of push-off you get when on land. You'll know by your breathing that you are getting a workout, but I also can tell by the feeling in my legs. Put your hand on your hamstring (back of your thigh) while running. You can feel it contracting as you move.

I have experimented with several deep-water running devices. One is a flotation belt. I was not happy with this "helper" because I felt that it prevented me from getting a good workout. This inexpensive device may help you stay afloat in the beginning, so give it a try. You can remove the belt when you are used to the activity.

I also tried solid-foam slippers. These relatively inexpensive slippers add resistance and buoyancy, but I found that while the belt makes it easier to stay afloat than do the slippers, I prefer the slippers. Both items are usually advertised in running magazines and are available in some sporting goods and specialty stores.

Here's a deep-water running workout to try. Run easy for 10 minutes. Do 10 to 15 one-minute intervals, running as hard as you can. Rest for 15 seconds between intervals by doing easy running. (Because you are in the water, your heart rate will not rise as high as when you

d, so you don't need as much recovery time.) Finish with a
e cool-down run.

Swimming. I am not a swimmer (which is one of the reasons I prefer deep-water running), but if you are, try this workout. Warm up by swimming a crawl for 10 to 12 pool lengths (for advanced swimmers, I'm assuming a pool length of 50 meters). Then swim 4 lengths at 80 to 85 percent of your maximum heart rate (MHR) and rest for 10 seconds. Repeat this 4-length segment a total of 6 to 10 times (10 to 15 minutes of hard effort). To cool down, swim 100 to 200 yards at an easy pace. After you swim the crawl, it's a good idea to stretch the chest and shoulders.

Cycling. Whether you bicycle outdoors or use a stationary bike indoors, invest in biking shorts that have padding. The first time someone suggested this to me, I laughed. I can use my running shorts, I thought. In the beginning, I sat on a towel, but eventually I did get biking shorts, and it makes a big difference. Now I don't get a sore seat at all.

Biking outdoors takes more time, but you do get the benefits of viewing the scenery and being outside. It's tempting to "cruise" on flat or downhill sections of road. But even on flat sections, you can control the difficulty of the exercise by shifting the bike into a higher gear. This will increase the resistance when you're pedaling and give you a better workout. Use a higher gear only on flat or downhill parts of the ride. When you bike with more resistance, especially uphill, you won't cycle as long, and you'll put more stress on your joints and increase your chances of getting injured.

Runners especially need to cycle with the pedals spinning above 85 revolutions per minute (rpm). Otherwise, they'll be working the quadriceps too hard. That's why they may benefit more from using a stationary bike, which allows them to pedal at a higher rpm more consistently. Most stationary bikes have an electronic display that gives an automatic rpm readout.

Cross-country skiing. For runners, I am most enthusiastic about cross-country ski machines. These machines most closely duplicate the running motion and actually provide even better fitness than running because they work both the upper and lower body. In addition, a cross-country trainer saves the legs from pounding. Initially, the machine may feel awkward, but after a few sessions, you'll get the hang of it. You can try out a machine at most gyms or sporting goods stores. Having a machine at home is an excellent option for the busy exerciser. I use mine two or three times a week.

Here's a good cross-country workout: Set the machine on easy to start (the handles and skis are at less resistance). Ski for 10 minutes to warm up, then increase the resistance in the arms and legs until your effort feels equivalent to a sustained run (70 to 80 percent of MHR). To make the effort a bit more rigorous, set the skis at a slight incline. Ski like that for 30 minutes. Cool down with an easy 10 minutes. If this is a bit too long, cut the sustained workout down to 20 minutes.

Skating. Looking to make your exercise fun? In-line skating may be great for you, although when I attempted it, I spent too much energy trying not to fall down. I prefer to ice-skate. I remember a day at Rockefeller Center in New York City when I ice-skated with my brother Jan right before the New York City Marathon in 1980. My husband was so angry at me! "You could have fallen and hurt yourself," he scolded. But I was young and fearless. What's more, the next day I set a world record in the marathon.

Jumping rope. This activity gets high marks for helping to build cardiovascular endurance, coordination, agility, and speed. It's also very convenient. Jumping rope works the upper and lower body and burns a lot of calories. But it also can be very taxing. Take it easy and don't get discouraged, especially in the beginning. Start with a short workout until you become accustomed to the exercise—and don't forget to warn any downstairs neighbors!

Make sure that the rope is the proper length (the handles should just touch your armpits when you're standing on the rope) and the handles are comfortable to hold. Warm up by lightly skipping rope or jogging in place. Wear supportive shoes and jump on a rug, the lawn, or a wooden floor. Concrete is too hard. Maintain good form: an erect posture, minimal swinging of the rope with the arms (concentrate on using just your wrists, not your entire arms), with your feet coming off the floor just enough to clear the rope.

Try any or all of the following routines, repeated as few or as many times as you wish.

> ↪ **Jump using alternate feet (like skipping). Start at moderate intensity (80 percent of MHR) and jump for 1-minute segments for a total of 5 or 6 minutes. Rest (by walking around) for 30 seconds between segments.**
> ↪ **Count while jumping (start with sets of 25 to 50).**
> ↪ **Move up to a higher intensity (85 to 90 percent of MHR). Jump for 10 seconds; rest for 30 seconds; jump for 20 seconds; rest for 20 seconds; jump for 30 seconds; rest for 10 seconds. You may add two-footed jumping and vary the time and intensity of any segment.**

Once you get the hang of jumping rope, you can invent your own workout and try various jumping and skipping steps. Remember to cool down and stretch after your workout. Jump at an intensity of at least 70 percent of MHR during the workout.

Stair climbing. If you don't have access to a stair-climbing machine, find a hotel, office building, apartment complex, or stadium with at least 50 steps. Begin by walking or, if you are warmed up and fit enough, running one step at a time. Swing your arms with the running motion to power yourself. Do not use handrails. If you are fatigued, slow down and walk or stop.

You can vary your stair climbing depending on your fitness level and the number of flights of stairs. For a sprint, keep your posture erect, with a gentle forward lean. Remember to cool down between sets by slowly walking back down or walking back and forth on the landings between flights.

Following is a workout I did many years ago in what was then the tallest building in Oslo. At about 10 floors, I began to take the steps two at a time for about 5 floors. Then, after cutting back to an easy walk of one step at a time for 2 floors, I did the hardest segment: three steps at a time for 5 floors.

Box stepping. Use a box or stair 8 to 16 inches in hei ..y higher, and you risk putting too much stress on your knees). Use only one-foot-at-a-time steps (that is, up with the right foot, joined by the left; down with the right foot, joined by the left) per set. As you do the steps, swing your arms in a running motion and keep an upright posture. Warm up by stepping at an easy pace or jogging in place for 5 to 10 minutes. Then try intervals: Walk hard for 1 minute, then easy for 30 seconds, repeating this segment 10 to 20 times depending on your conditioning. To cool down, just step slower or walk or jog.

Fitness for the Fast-Paced

As I mentioned earlier, cross-training is highly flexible and can be easily adapted to whatever time you have. If you have a busy schedule, consider these options to make the most of your fitness time.

Make your activities seasonal. Since land running is often more uncomfortable in the heat and humidity, alternate with deep-water running in the summer. In the winter, try cross-country skiing, hiking in the snow, or snowshoeing.

Cross-train at home. You don't have to go to a gym to cross-train. At home, try jumping rope or using exercise videos. These can provide hard bouts of exercise. For a cool-down, you can walk it off or turn up the volume and dance to the music.

Get the entire family involved. Activities such as tennis, basketball, and soccer are great cross-training activities not only because they give you excellent exercise but also because you can do them with your family. Don't underestimate the power of playing family games. Many people get a great workout by trying to keep up with the kids.

Look for time-savers. If you have a busy schedule, look for ways to save time in other activities and to combine those activities with a workout. Bring your work clothes to the health club. Bike, walk, or skate to your errands. Instead of sitting down for a business or social meeting, chat during a walk or run. The more you look for these time-saving opportunities, the more you'll find.

Fitting In Fitness

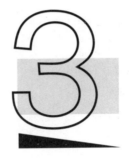

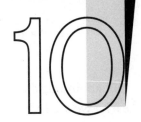

The Fitness Lifestyle
Advice for the Busy Exerciser

I understand the life of a busy exerciser because I live it every day. Like most people, my day is filled with appointments and obligations. I'm very honest with myself. I know that if I don't get my exercise done in the morning, I won't get it done at all. On a typical day, I may have scheduled an 8:00 A.M. breakfast meeting. That means I must leave the house by about 7:15. If it's a busy day, I may have other business or meetings in the city during the afternoon. So I'm out the door to run, walk, or bike by 5:30 A.M.

Very often, between obligations, I use the lunch hour for a social visit. I suppose I could fit in exercise then, but I don't like to rush when I work out, so it isn't worth it to me.

When I get home in the late afternoon or early evening after a day of being "up on my toes" (my expression for my type of work stress) all day, I'm very tired. I usually shop for groceries on the way home and then must attend to telephone messages and faxes and make calls to the United States. The afternoon also is a hectic time of phone calls for Jack, my morning exercise partner, because his business is largely done overseas. By the dinner hour, we are done in. We eat at home and talk about our day. We almost never go out. Because our day begins so early, we are in bed by 9 P.M.

I realize that your life may be very different from mine. For one thing, I don't have children to shuttle to soccer practice or other activities. If you have teenagers, for instance, they may not get home until 7:30 P.M. By the time you've eaten and visited a bit, perhaps caught up on chores, and gotten things ready for the next day, it's well past 9:00. But no matter what your situation, wise planning is required to make exercise possible.

Most exercisers work out three or four times a week. If you exercise on the weekends, you need to plan for only two other days during the week. Over the years, I have heard all the excuses for not exercising. Everything from not having the right shoes to workplaces that lack shower and training facilities. But most people say that they just don't have enough time. When it comes to exercise, it seems, most people don't like to plan; they prefer to go with the flow. But if you ever hope to stick with a program, you must make exercise a priority. Exercising regularly has nothing to do with athletic ability. It has everything to do with dedication and discipline.

There is a woman in my athletic club in Oslo whom I have known since she was 18, when it was clear that she was a very talented 800-meter runner. Now she is 30 years old, a mother of two, and unhappy about being overweight. She wants to get back in shape, but she is the kind of runner who has to have everything perfect. The weather has to be good, everything must be well organized, and she must be in the right mood. She was always that way, even as a young competitor. As an elite athlete, she had the talent but not the character or the dedication. She is the kind of person I call "soft."

By contrast, the former prime minister of Norway, Gro Harlem Brundtland, managed to train for and complete the Grete Waitz Run while still in office. President Bill Clinton also is an avid runner who, according to friends of mine who have trained with him, keeps a very good pace. It seems to me that if heads of state can find time to exercise, the rest of us surely can.

When to Work Out

Every time of day has its advantages. You simply have to balance your schedule and your style with the various possibilities. Because I travel a lot and sometimes have an erratic lifestyle, I like to work out first thing in the morning, between 5:00 and 5:30 A.M. (Even in my competitive days, I did my first workout at this time.) Unless you have a health club in your home, there is very little you can do at this hour except bike, walk, or run. I am happy with any of those options. I also am able to work out at my health club because it opens very early in the morning.

The advantage of early-morning exercise is that there is little to distract you. There is not nearly as much going on at 6:00 A.M. as there is at 6:00 P.M. According to surveys I've read, people who exercise in the morning tend to stick to it more than those who work out at other times of the day.

There is one disadvantage to an early-morning workout, however. Many people have a hard time dragging themselves out of bed. And who can just jump up and run? It's best to give yourself at least 20 minutes to wake up and get going. Start with coffee or juice if you wish. Wake up the body by making the bed or doing other chores. And ease into your exercise by doing the first 5 to 10 minutes at a slower pace.

The advantages of exercising in the afternoon or early evening are physical. The body temperature is higher then, and the muscles and joints are more flexible. But if you've had a long, hard day, you may not be able to use this physical advantage, as you may be too tired.

Beware of working out too late in the evening, as you may have a hard time getting to sleep. After exercise, the body is revved up. Working out late also may cause you to delay eating until too close to bedtime. This combination of exercise and a full stomach may keep you awake. I always had a hard time sleeping after an evening, or even an afternoon, race because I was wired mentally and physically. Although I was tired from the neck down, I was working overtime from the neck up. These days, I'm the same way after doing a clinic or a speech.

From my past experience of training twice a day, I would say that the best time physiologically is midafternoon from 3:00 to 4:00 P.M. But workouts at this hour are impractical for many, if not most, people. If you arrange to work out at this time even though it means upsetting your normal schedule, you probably aren't integrating exercise too well into your lifestyle.

Once you settle on the best time of day for exercise, do you have to stick with that time? The difficulty in changing workout times is probably both physiological and psychological. After all, we are creatures of habit, and we do seem to have an internal clock. I feel out of sync if I run at any other time than what I am used to. If I try to change times, my body feels as if it is rebelling. I feel heavy-legged and sluggish, and because I am used to running in the early morning before eating, I can sense an earlier meal sloshing around in my stomach. If you anticipate a change in exercise time, plan your meals in advance. You should wait at least 1 to 2 hours after a snack, 3 hours after a small meal, and longer after a larger one.

There is a great benefit to being flexible about your exercise time. With a busy lifestyle, it's nice to be able to exercise whenever you can fit it in. But I think there are great advantages to working out at the same time every day. The legendary Villanova University track coach Jumbo Elliott used to tell his runners, "Live like a clock." Eat the same, run the same, and sleep the same.

Finding the Time to Train

In Norway we say, "The perception of a problem is always relative." A plane reservation and my husband serve as an example. If we are scheduled to fly early in the morning, Jack will easily sacrifice a workout. "I can do this, but I can't do that," he will say. But I tell him, if we organize our time, we can do both. We pack all the gear the night before the trip. The next morning, we get up half an hour earlier than usual. We finish our run and put the dirty clothes in a plastic bag. We never make breakfast at home but pack a bagel and banana to bring along or eat at the airport. As for fatigue, we can always sleep on the plane. Successful exercise is all in the planning. As the saying goes, "Where there's a will, there's a way."

See solutions instead of obstacles. Instead of dwelling on why you can't work out on an upcoming busy day, focus on a creative way to make your exercise happen.

Plan ahead. You don't have to work out on very busy days, but it may make a positive difference when you can. Visualize and organize your day to fit in that morning exercise session. If I am facing a very big day, I make sure the night before that I have both my training gear and my work clothes already laid out, the alarm set a few minutes earlier than usual, and the papers or materials for the next day's work packed.

Use exercise for transportation. Take advantage of good weather. Particularly in the summer, the streets are full of bikers of every size and shape. Again, planning is key. If you want to run, walk, or bike to a destination, pack with you (or store ahead of time) a change of clothes and supplies.

Be creative. I once saw a group of six women pushing babies in strollers in New York City's Central Park. They congregated at the bottom of a hill and, after warming up, pushed the strollers up the hill, then chatted as they walked back down for recovery. They did this over and over again. It was a rigorous workout and a pleasant social event as well. My friends in Norway often go to the track to exercise. Their children play with sand toys in the long jump pit while they circle the track doing intervals.

Make it a family affair. When my nephews were young, I involved them in my training. While I ran, one would time me while the other recorded those times in a book. Then I would tell them that it was their turn, and they would run. When they were six and eight years old, I brought them to New York City for a race I was running. I also took them to a running camp.

Organize groups. Whether it's on the job or with a group of stay-at-home moms, build a program around a convenient time and situation.

Bring along washing supplies. For a light jog or other exercise that will end away from home, carry a few supplies, such as a small towel, soap, and deodorant, in a lightweight backpack. Then you can easily wash up in a sink at your destination. I've done this many times.

Pack a snack. I always take a drink and a banana if I won't be working out at home. This serves as a postworkout snack and helps me avoid buying the junk food that's usually available.

Schedule your workouts. Consider your training as important as your other appointments. I always schedule appointments around my workout times and am firm about not bumping my exercise. I try to suggest times that I know won't interfere with my workouts.

Tailor the exercise to the place and time. If running or walking is difficult because of bad weather or an inconvenient location, plan an indoor activity such as swimming or riding a stationary bike. If no facility is available, try jumping rope or box stepping. (For more information on these activities, see chapter 9.)

Making the Commitment

My exercise prescription is user-friendly. It is time-efficient, sensible, doable, and, once the habit is developed, easy to maintain. Running or walking is the least time-consuming and least expensive form of exercise. Running is my number one sport, but I know it's not for everyone. It's easy and one of the most efficient activities in terms of getting in shape and burning calories. I realize that it is not so easy to do this activity at home, for example, because a treadmill is very expensive. That's why I also recommend using a stationary bike or cross-country ski machine as an alternative.

Rodale Press, publisher of *Prevention* and *Men's Health* magazines, has discovered that most of these magazines' readers are not health club members. Many people are too busy to use a health club, or they feel intimidated if they don't know how to use the equipment. My husband, Jack, for example, doesn't know how to use the machines and doesn't like to ask for help. One of the biggest hurdles for people

Health Club Happiness

Many people are motivated by joining a health club or fitness center. I chose my health club in Gainesville, Florida, first and foremost because it opens very early in the morning, when I like to work out. I go there mostly to bike, so having good stationary bikes is important to me as well. Good air-conditioning and cleanliness also influenced my decision. Here are some tips to help you find the right health club.

Make sure you're getting value. A health club membership can cost $400 to $600 a year. Unless you're going to use the facility at least three times a week, it's probably not worth your money.

Give it a trial run. Most clubs have a free test hour. Try to get to know as much of the equipment and as many of the programs as you can before joining.

Check the air quality. People often overlook the importance of good air circulation. When doing your trial workout, if you feel uncharacteristically out of breath or you begin sweating early or profusely, perhaps the facility is not well ventilated.

Shop around. Don't be fooled by ads that claim exercise is easy, always fun, and inexpensive and that as soon as you get your membership, you'll see a change.

Get a feel for the atmosphere. You have to feel comfortable and like the surroundings so that you'll look forward to going. If, for instance, you're in your fifties, you may not like it if the majority of clients are in their twenties.

Look into other benefits. Most clubs have classes in aerobics, dancing, and yoga. If you are interested in these other forms of exercise, check out the kind of training conditions—space, type of floor, and ventilation—the club offers.

Check the locker rooms. They should be clean and spacious. Many clubs have a locker room attendant, which is a nice benefit.

Meet the staff. They should be professional, available, and inspirational. Ask members of the club about the staff. Check the certification of all trainers and instructors.

Visit during your exercise times. Before you sign up, find out the conditions during the hours when you might train. Is there a long wait on the most popular machines, such as treadmills and stair climbers?

who are unfit is embarrassment. Often people say, "When I get in better shape, I'm going to join a health club."

Health clubs can, however, be very effective. You may be inspired and motivated by the qualified coaching, helpful information, and socializing that these clubs offer.

In the old days, when I was competing and the fitness boom was at its peak, it never occurred to most of us to vary our forms of exercise. Running was all I did. Later, when triathlons became popular, the idea of multisport participation took hold, and it has never let go.

I emphasize variety to all exercisers. If fitness and health are your goals, once you get in decent shape, you can avoid injury and burnout by cross-training (see chapter 9). If you enjoy running, build a fitness base (see the beginning program in chapter 4), then try biking or swimming. By doing a variety of sports, you will find out what you like best and what works for you. Then you can develop that activity. Often I meet injured runners who take up biking, then try participating in duathlons—biking and running competitions.

Sporadic Exercisers

Most of the people I meet are sporadic exercisers. They begin with enthusiasm and the desire to work out, but some event, such as the holidays, causes them to fall off the wagon. Regular exercisers, as I call them, get back on their programs after these interruptions, but sporadic exercisers don't. Once these people break the exercise routine, they damage a positive and important life pattern. That's because it is often difficult for people in this situation to see a lapse as temporary. It is like the dieter who has one piece of cake, curses the fact that the diet is broken, and then turns around and eats the entire cake. Sporadic exercisers often start exercising again when they feel lousy and out of shape. Unfortunately, they see exercise as a kind of temporary, rather negative endeavor, as opposed to a permanent, positive activity. They're just setting themselves up to break the exercise routine again.

What is the difference between a sporadic and a regular exerciser? Minimally, those who stop exercising for three weeks or longer, three to five times a year, are sporadic exercisers. A regular exerciser might take off for three to four weeks once a year, but that isn't a recurring event.

11

On the Job
Making It Work

Work is work, even if your job is also your passion. After a decade of a tense, work-and-run schedule, I quit my teaching job to run full-time. At first I thought, how nice not to have to go to work. As much as I loved running, however, it wasn't long before I realized that running, too, is a job. Sometimes before I went out to train, I would leave a note for my husband that said, "I've gone to work. Be back in a couple of hours."

No matter what your job, if you're trying to combine it with exercise, your day is likely very full. When I was teaching and training twice a day, everything had to be managed according to the clock. I couldn't have survived without scheduling every minute. I lived as if I had a stopwatch in my hand. Breakfast was exactly 10 minutes. One extra minute, and I'd miss my bus or train. Every piece of clothing, every book or bag, had to be laid out the night before.

My teaching job entailed 3 hours of commuting every day. Even though there were some breaks in the school day, those weren't feasible times for me to train. (That's where most exercisers are luckier. What I was doing then was beyond exercise and couldn't be done anywhere, at any time.) My habit of early-morning running became entrenched during those years. There was no other way. I also ran again when I got home from work.

I can't say that I enjoyed my work/running schedule (although I did enjoy each task individually), but I was prepared to do what it took to be a world-class runner. At the same time, I needed to do my job. In those years, even the world's best runners weren't making a living at the sport. Besides, I had been trained to do both things.

Looking back, I don't know how I survived those years. At the time, I didn't think about the situation, but I always felt the tension in the pit of my stomach. There were days that I was so tired, I would look at the pile of training clothes awaiting me and burst out crying. But I always put on the gear and went out to run. And I always felt better afterward.

At the very least, this dual life gave me some balance. Work kept my mind off worrying about running and prevented me from putting too much focus on it. What's more, this schedule demonstrated not only my willpower but also my toughness, determination, and discipline. When you successfully blend your work life and exercise, you'll find these qualities in yourself as well.

I firmly believe that no mountain is too high if you really want to get to the top. This is a crucial point and the basic theme of this chapter. (In fact, it is the theme of the entire book.) As in every aspect of a busy person's life, you need willpower and motivation. When you find these qualities, they will help you to make the necessary compromises or sacrifices. Fitting exercise into any schedule, no matter how difficult, is the ultimate statement of how important your health and well-being are to you.

Why the Workplace?

As I emphasize throughout the book, I believe that morning exercise is best. My friend Barbara Paddock, vice president and director of sports marketing for Chase Manhattan Bank, agrees. She works out every morning because "once I'm in the office, I'm committed. I stay there." She makes a morning running date with another corporate friend. "If I don't have the commitment to meet someone, I just roll over and go back to sleep." Not only does her date get her out the door, but their chats help her to work out problems.

There are some benefits to combining your work and exercise, though. After all, work is where you spend most of your day. It can be very convenient to take your sneakers out of your desk drawer and just go do it. You don't have to waste any time traveling long distances to a gym; you don't have to drag yourself out of bed in the early hours of the morning or work out in the dark. You can do it by yourself or forge new bonds by finding friends and co-workers with whom you can share your exercise.

Here are some tips on successfully blending both your exercise and work life.

Work out to or from work. Try to run, walk, or bike to work. That's what we do in Norway. It's an easy way to integrate fitness into your life, and you can kill two birds with one stone.

Make it social. In Norway, we also have organized neighborhood and corporate team activities, such as running, track and field, team handball, and soccer. In the United States, you can join softball and basketball teams, walking groups, and many other activities.

Try lunchtime workouts. Walking is one activity that you can do without showering (I hope!).

Find a gym or health club nearby. If you don't need all the facilities and just want locker and shower privileges, check out a partial membership.

Job-share. If possible, create a cooperative relationship with a fellow worker that allows you the time and opportunity to exercise during the most convenient part of the workday.

Find free exercise. Walk up and down flights of stairs or walk the hallways of your workplace for some exercise. If it's fitness you want, this may not work. But if you want to burn some extra calories, there's bound to be plenty of free exercise in the workplace.

Walk and talk. Do business over exercise rather than over meals. I discovered this approach while visiting the Motorola Corporation in Chicago. There is a 1.5-mile exercise course nearby, and a top company executive often told his associates, "I need some exercise. You probably do, too. We'll do this meeting walking." When the boss suggests something, you don't say no!

Look into flextime. If being on the job from nine to five isn't a requirement, rearrange your day to accommodate your exercise. I have friends who go to work in the late morning after exercising, then stay until late evening.

The Chase Corporate Challenge

Since 1980, I have been deeply involved with the Chase Corporate Challenge, serving as spokesperson and attending many of its 3.5-mile races. The Corporate Challenge began in 1977 with 200 participants from 50 companies in New York City. It has grown to 150,000 participants from 6,000 companies who compete in 17 cities and 3 countries, making it the largest corporate sporting event in the world. Barbara Paddock, an executive at Chase, is a committed runner who has completed two marathons. She has helped nurture and develop the Corporate Challenge since its beginning. I asked her why she feels the event has grown so astoundingly.

"Everybody in corporate America is trying to integrate health and fitness into their work lives," Paddock says. "The health movement of the 1970s and 1980s got people conscious of exercising, and the easiest way to integrate it into their lives is at the workplace. Also, with mergers and other developments, the workload is more stressful. People have to work harder and perform better. While the demands are greater, there is also a need to watch out for oneself in terms of health and well-being."

Paddock also attributes the event's success to the fact that it's about more than fitness; it's about having a good time on the job. "The Corporate Challenge includes seasoned runners, but the greater majority are casual joggers, walkers, and bikers," she notes. "We created the Corporate Challenge for serious runners, but we also created it for an atmosphere of fun. We are adamant about keeping it a one-night, weeknight event. It isn't [meant] to cut into weekend family time."

Who are these people who successfully fit fitness into the workplace? They are capable, ambitious, can-do individuals. "The great majority are middle to upper management," Paddock says. "In addition to those established in business, there are young, up-and-coming people. In fact, those Corporate Challenge participants in the 1970s who were in training programs are now managing directors." It is these people—clearly successful in many aspects of life—who bring the fitness message back to their companies. "We are providing the ingredients," Paddock says, "but all these capable workers, a very enthusiastic bunch of people, are motivating others."

The Corporate Challenge shows some of the expected and unexpected benefits of on-the-job fitness programs. Many of the companies that participate also sponsor health and fitness clinics and lunch-hour fitness programs, and their newsletters feature both Corporate Challenge entry information and training tips. "The beauty of the event is that it's not only about exercise," Paddock says. "I think we've created something beyond that: camaraderie. People design team uniforms and banners; they book restaurants and have parties. Many come out just to cheer. They are together in a unique atmosphere outside the office. And even those in the company who don't participate are aware of the event."

Model Companies

Over the years, I have had the opportunity to visit various companies to promote fitness. Companies with organized fitness programs are much more likely to have employees who are dedicated and disciplined when it comes to exercising. The ideal situation is on-the-job support, with an exercise and fitness program built and conducted by experts. It is probably unrealistic to expect every company and employer to provide these benefits. But on-the-job fitness need not be so formal.

Fitness Facts

The following facts are from a brochure about the economic impact of work site health promotion published by American Corporate Health Programs of Exton, Pennsylvania.

↳ An 18-month study by General Electric reported on a 38 percent decrease in health care costs for fitness program members compared with a 21 percent increase for nonmembers.

↳ Job performance was strongly correlated with exercise adherence in a study of 3,231 white-collar workers. Those who received the highest performance ratings from supervisors also were the most likely to adhere to exercise programs.

↳ Fitness and health promotion programs are associated with reducing employee absenteeism. DuPont reduced absenteeism by 47.5 percent over six years after instituting a fitness program.

↳ The Dallas Police Department noted a 39 percent increase in commendations after a fitness/lifestyle program was introduced to officers.

↳ In a nine-month analysis of decision-making capabilities, exercisers showed a distinct advantage—a 70 percent greater performance—over nonexercisers.

↳ Control Data credited its wellness program with saving the company $1.8 million in reduced medical claims.

Again, I use Norway as an example. Many employees take the initiative to organize their own programs. Often they use space in a spare room or the basement. The program is run by one or two employee volunteers. Some companies, such as *KK,* the largest women's magazine in Norway, conduct programs before work. Others, such as Manpower, an international company with a branch in Norway, have informal post-work exercise programs. These programs may not be organized in a traditional sense, but at least exercise happens.

A small number of forward-looking companies in the United States have developed ideal on-the-job programs. One of the most impressive programs is run by Rodale Press, which has been widely recognized by professional health groups for its efforts in this area. Of course, it only makes sense that the publisher of health and fitness magazines and books should be a role model.

When I first went to visit Rodale headquarters in Emmaus, Pennsylvania, I ran into Budd Coates, a 2:13 marathoner and a top runner who had competed in my day. Sixteen years ago, Coates developed Rodale's fitness program. Today, as work site health promotion manager, he oversees programs that include a health and fitness center (also available to the families of participating employees) with a full array of aerobic and weight equipment, nutrition classes, incentive awards, golf and tennis leagues, and classes in everything from yoga and scuba diving to fly-fishing and walking. Rodale also has an in-house health educator and regular health screenings for employees. All of Rodale's cafeterias feature healthy and delicious food. (You'll never see burgers and fries on the menu.) Perhaps the most impressive fact is that a remarkable 75 percent of the company's employees take advantage of the fitness program.

Not everyone can work at a company like Rodale, but Coates believes that everyone can bring some element of exercise and fitness to the job. He offers the following suggestions to get fitness going in the workplace.

Get involved. If things are done in a positive way and employees get involved, you'll get attention sooner or later.

Be a can-do, positive person. Support rather than condemn. If the cafeteria food is unhealthy, don't just complain; offer concrete suggestions to improve the menu. Sign up for an event like the Chase Corporate Challenge. Take pictures of workers at the event and send them to the boss with an upbeat, positive message.

Find or develop a group event. Coed softball teams are popular, and walking groups are convenient. Rodale charters two buses every year for the 100 workers who participate in the Chase Corporate Challenge. Rodale also rents out an Italian restaurant for a postrace party. The only rules for participating in the race are that you have to be able to run or walk the 3.5-mile distance and you have to be on time for work the next day. Managers at Rodale report that Corporate Challenge employees usually come in early the next day—often to brag about their accomplishments!

Use word of mouth, company newsletters, memos, and e-mail. Get your message out in as many ways as possible. If you need walking or running partners, for instance, post the date and time on e-mail.

Can Coates's suggestions for marshaling support in the workplace be successful? "We've done it here," he relates. "In 1981, two of us ran the Boston Marathon with Rodale Press logos we ironed on our singlets. The crowds were cheering support all along the way, telling us they read our publications. We were telling the story in the company cafeteria and didn't realize that sitting right behind us was Bob Rodale, the chairman of the board. He was so impressed by what he overheard that he said from that date on, anyone who qualified for the Boston Marathon got the Monday of the race off in order to run, and the hotel and entry fee would be paid for by the company. It was also at that time that we started the Fitness Center. One of our employees renamed it the Energy Center. That's because it takes energy to get there, and the result of exercising is that you get more energy."

Not All Jobs Are in the Office

Many jobs—from sales and service professions to teaching school—are not done in an office, nor do all employees work for corporations. Initiative and creativity are necessary to fit exercise into these jobs. Parenting also is a job, and being with children offers some excellent ways to integrate fitness into your life. In Norway, one forum for adult exercise is the sports club (see chapter 1). Although these clubs traditionally focus on youth sports (I joined my club as a child), in the past 20 years they also have incorporated adult fitness. Instead of sitting around waiting for the kids, parents now use that time to participate in their own exercise activities. Fitting in exercise in these ways can lead to many other opportunities, from informal parent baby-sitting co-ops to school-based support programs.

Having been a teacher myself, I think it would be great to launch an exercise program that includes both students and teachers. One such program, created by the New York Road Runners Club, is Run Across America. (For a booklet on how to implement this program in your school or youth group, send a self-addressed stamped envelope with 55 cents postage to Run Across America, c/o NYRRC, 9 East 89th Street, New York, NY 10128.) One New York City middle school teacher has twice-weekly after-school running groups. She singles out a number of girls to train with her on weekends in preparation for the Advil Mini-Marathon 10-K (6.2 miles) for women, a race I won five times.

Other jobs require other methods. One runner I know, a chef by profession, has a rather long commute, including a ferry ride. He runs to and from the ferry. Other work challenges require a creative approach. If you own a shop or work in a small business, one solution might be to hire inexpensive lunchtime or after-school help while you take an hour off to exercise. Certain jobs present challenges other than time. If you're on your feet all day at work, adding weight-bearing exercise can be stressful. You might want to build your fitness around swimming. If you want to include running or walking, save it for your days off.

When the Going Gets Tough

Throughout this book, I have acknowledged many of the difficulties busy people face in fitting in exercise. Perhaps no area is more difficult to negotiate than that of a stressful work life. But many of the problems I've found include self-motivation, time management, and personal priorities—not the job itself.

Barbara Paddock is a good example. Although she has been a runner since 1974, she recently stopped exercising for a year and a half because of the stress of a bank merger, which put her job in jeopardy. "The stress and job uncertainty meant I was working all day and all night. Instead of running, I would go to bed," she says. Paddock began to experience an array of physical problems, which she now realizes were related to stress. "I was more committed to the office than I was to myself. I had to do something for me." Being fit is important "to keep your sense of self," Paddock says. She concludes that without the de-stressing of exercise time, workers cannot meet the demands of the job and maintain the high standards that are required in today's business and corporate climate.

Another acquaintance illustrates the importance of setting priorities. She is a 53-year-old social worker and family counselor, whose job stress is compounded by a significant number of daily crises. Her job, coupled with her own family's needs (she helps care for her parents and has three grown children who are very much a part of her life), creates plenty of stress. For years she found it difficult to fit in her exercise. There was always someone who needed her time, always a reason to put off her workout. Then her doctor prescribed an exercise program for her. She was, in a sense, ordered to do it.

Setting aside at least 20 minutes a day for walking has been much less of a physical effort than a psychological one. She has taken various steps to ensure that she keeps these "appointments" with herself. First, she bought a treadmill to use in bad weather or when it is dark. Then, although her new exercise program had no particular relevance to her co-workers, she reinforced her resolve by announcing it during a staff meeting. Finally, she turned to a neighborhood friend—a successful athlete with informal coaching experience—for help. He guided her in creating a program. More important, he is available to talk and, when necessary, walk with her.

At some point, you may be forced to make unexpected decisions about your lifestyle and priorities. That was the case in my career. I had been teaching for two years when I decided I was probably going to retire from competitive running. I made this decision for two reasons. First, I felt I had realized my potential as a track runner. If women had been allowed to run longer distances in international competition, perhaps my decision would have been different. (When I competed, 1500 meters was the longest race for women in the Olympic Games. Women also competed in the 3000 meters, though not in the Olympics. Today women run a full range of longer distances, including the marathon.)

Second, I was tired. In the beginning, I was so motivated that I could manage it all. But after a few years of working and training, the fatigue had a cumulative effect. I wondered whether I should keep putting myself through this for the limited opportunities I had on the track. Then, in 1978, I ran a marathon, and it turned my life around.

Shortly after I set a world record in that first marathon, the offers and invitations to run other events began to pour in. I tried very hard to schedule my running events around my teaching job. When I couldn't, I used sick days, paid time off, and substitutes. Nevertheless, by 1980, the conflict between work and running was becoming too great. The headmaster asked me to make a decision: Devote more time to the job or quit. I felt guilty about taking days off and was frustrated by the difficulty of doing both tasks. I didn't like the fact that sometimes I'd be so tired, I'd find myself teaching a physical education class while sitting on a bench and blowing my whistle instead of participating as I usually did.

The choice was not an easy one. I would be going from something very secure (my monthly income from teaching) to something very insecure (supporting myself by running). Jack was an accountant, but we couldn't live on his salary. In those days, the money for runners wasn't great, and it certainly wasn't guaranteed or regular. What if I got ill or injured? As the Norwegian saying goes, should I put all my eggs in one hat?

I decided to take a one-year leave of absence from my teaching job. Finally, I had time to rest between workouts. I could pay attention to my home and the rest of my life. I could train away from the Norwegian winters. And as my success on the roads grew, I knew there was no going back.

Did I miss teaching? I didn't miss disciplining teenagers, but I did miss the craft of teaching. I still do. That is why, in my way, I feel I have come back to it today. When I speak to groups and work with people, I use my skills as a teacher. When asked to do a clinic or give a speech, I much prefer to educate than to talk about myself. In my earlier days, I taught Norwegian, history, geography, and physical education to grade school children. Now I teach health and fitness to people of all ages.

12

On the Road
Exercising Away from Home

Many busy people find themselves out and about a great deal of the time. That's the nature of being busy: you're not home much. In addition, you surely don't have the convenience of abundant free time—which would make it much easier and more comfortable to exercise. I have years of experience with fitting in exercise while traveling, but my first piece of advice is philosophical. It has to do with balance and expectations.

If you encounter a busy time or hectic situation, keep a sensible perspective. Exercise is a top priority for me, but if I can't work out, I don't. If you can't exercise for two or three days, you won't lose your fitness—and you're not going to gain 6 pounds either. In fact, time off from exercise can be an asset—it can help keep your routine fresh. As a dedicated exerciser, you will often come back to your workout program energized and refreshed after taking a break.

Although I really enjoy my exercise and don't like to give it up, sometimes I am forced to do so. I am almost always on the road. In addition to splitting my time between two countries, I travel around the world at least 10 percent of the time. I travel across time zones. I get tired. There may be no place to run or no facilities for me to cross-train. All kinds of things get in the way of exercise, many of which are beyond our control.

Having said that, I must add that you can fit in exercise on the road. Here are some of the things I do to help make it easier. Although the tips are related to long-distance travel, many of them apply to travel of any length of time or distance.

Take your exercise equipment with you. Pack lightweight items, such as a jump rope or elastic exercise band (used for resistance exercises), to help you get in a little training wherever you are.

Wear your running shoes. I always wear my running shoes while traveling. As a matter of fact, I wear running shoes nearly everywhere. I don't want to put any other kind of shoes on my feet unless I have to. If I need to wear dress shoes, I carry them in a bag and change right before (and again right after) my meeting or appointment. Running shoes are comfortable and convenient, and they also accommodate walking. They're especially comfortable when you travel by plane, since your feet tend to swell. Another reason I wear my sneakers to travel is if my luggage should get lost, I'll at least have my shoes to work out in. My other exercise gear is more easily replaced.

Do your own laundry. I carry just one exercise outfit on the road, but I also carry laundry soap. (If you can't find it in travel packs, just pack it yourself in a zipper-locked plastic bag.) Even in my competitive days, I washed out my own workout gear in hotel sinks. This clothing dries quickly and is ready to wear the next day.

Get a good travel agent. Find a travel agent who is sympathetic to your exercise needs, preferably one with experience in this area. A good travel agent can help you make reservations at hotels that have their own exercise facilities or that are near places where you can work out. If you make your own travel plans, look for a hotel close to a park, riverbank, or other area where you can run. Ask if the hotel has a health club and check to see if its hours are convenient for you.

Do drop in. Health clubs, especially those in major cities, often have drop-in rates. It never hurts to call and ask. If you belong to a health club that is part of a national chain, you may not even have to pay a drop-in fee. Some clubs, such as the YMCA and YWCA, also allow you to use branches in other places for free.

Be a flexible traveler. Choose an exercise activity that easily fits into the area where you are staying. If running isn't a good option, check out a local health club or rent a bike. Be creative. If there are a lot of hills nearby, walk or run them repeatedly. If the hotel has a staircase, try using it for exercise.

Take an active vacation. Take a vacation in a place that accommodates hiking, bicycling, horseback riding, or other physical activities. I know of some runners who jog from place to place. For families who like active vacations, check out sports camps or sports travel packages. For years I attended the adidas running camp in the northeastern United States and would often bring family members with me.

If you're on vacation, it's okay to lay low with your training. Don't let it interfere with your trip. Remember, sight-seeing often entails a lot of walking or other activities that qualify as exercise. Enjoying the vacation should be your first priority.

Travel Tips for Those on the Run

If your fitness plans revolve primarily around running and walking, you're at a definite advantage when you travel. After all, there aren't many places in the world where you can't do either one. But if you want to make your exercise safe, healthy, and enjoyable no matter where you are, here's some useful advice.

Run early. The best time to run or walk in a city is the early morning, when there is less traffic, fewer people are out and about, and there are fewer distractions in general.

Ask for directions. When you arrive at your destination, ask around for the best places to walk or run. Find out whether the hotel has a running map, and if so use it. This will help you see the sights better and avoid trouble. Several times I have found myself running in some not-so-nice parts of town.

Check the culture. Inquire about appropriate dress and other cultural traditions. Some cultures don't appreciate seeing people, especially women, in shorts and sleeveless tops.

Be prepared. No matter what exercise you enjoy, when you go out, take some sensible precautions. If you're going out alone, let someone know where you intend to run and about how long you will be gone—even if it means telling the hotel staff. Always carry some local currency with you. You may need it for an emergency telephone call, transportation, or even a drink. Also be sure to carry some identification. I take my room key, which has the name of the hotel on it.

Don't get lost. It's easy to fall into the trap of running the way you do at home—on automatic pilot. But you need to be more attentive in strange surroundings. More than once I have forgotten what hotel room I was in and have walked the halls whispering Jack's name, hoping for one of the identical doors to open. Outside, don't be ashamed to ask for directions. Whereas Jack prefers to try to negotiate a route himself (even if it means running in circles), I'm more apt to ask for help. I'm not good with directions, especially in a strange place, so I never try to figure out the way myself.

Be adventurous. Don't always believe what you hear about places not being safe for running or walking. New York City has a bad reputation, but you can find people out running and walking at any hour. One morning a police car's loudspeaker greeted me with the words "Good morning, Grete." It was a nice touch, and it made me feel secure.

13

Clothes and Shoes
They've Come a Long Way

This chapter was written with the assistance of Chris Jones, an all-around athlete and product line manager for running apparel for adidas USA. Chris worked in retail sales for many years.

Those of us who are longtime exercisers and athletes were pioneers in the area of workout gear. No wonder I was able to develop my running strength: I was always carrying a load of bulky clothing with me as I ran. As for my early shoes, it's amazing that I was never seriously injured. The shoes I wore for my first marathon in 1978 were so bad by today's standards that now I wouldn't even wear them to walk to the mailbox. Over the past 25 years, the development of exercise equipment has been revolutionary.

Today we all benefit from the technological advances made in exercise gear. An increasingly active population spurred many of these advances. As a representative and spokesperson for adidas since 1980, I have been in the vanguard of testing various equipment. In addition to representing adidas at a variety of worldwide events and races, my work for the company includes experimenting with, and providing feedback on, every type of shoe and exercise wear available.

When purchasing workout clothing, the busy exerciser must look for versatility and efficiency. This is true not only in regard to the usefulness of the gear itself, but also in shopping for it.

Buying What's Best for You

The first thing to know about clothing is that it pays to invest in gear made of technologically advanced fabrics. You can still exercise in baggy old sweats, but if you are a busy person, you want to make your exercise time count. You will exercise more efficiently, comfortably, and safely if you have the proper gear. Here are three important rules to keep in mind when shopping for gear.

Think layers. Buying for versatility means that you should go for multiple lighter-weight layers as opposed to one heavy layer. The key term these days is *moisture management*, also called *wicking*. This refers to the material's ability to pull perspiration away from the body, thus spreading the moisture out so that it dries quickly.

Stay away from cotton. "It feels great against the skin," Jones says, "and it's fine in perfect weather (mild and windless), but because cotton holds moisture, even the slightest breeze against your wet skin will give you a chill." For indoor aerobic exercise, and for most outdoor workouts, wear moisture management clothing made of synthetics (basically polyester and nylon).

Expensive is not always better. A higher price means more features, but they may not be the ones you need. This is important, particularly if the added features make the equipment heavier or bulkier.

Jones gives the following tips on buying exercise gear.

Shop in specialty stores or quality sporting goods stores. These stores are my personal preference because they promote their sports and the community, but if you know what you're looking for, you can probably find the gear cheaper in other stores.

Beware of big outlets. They usually don't have a wide selection of technical gear, as they are not sport specific, and they generally don't have very knowledgeable staff. It is often difficult to find the items you want or the sales help you need. Especially for a busy person, the few dollars you might save are probably not worth the time you'll spend hunting around for what you need.

Be prepared to help. For the best service, give the salespeople some information about the activity you do, including where (surface, weather and wind conditions) and how much you do it. In addition, determine whether you are genetically a "warm" or "cool" person. I tend to be cool, which means I wear more clothing. Others warm up quickly and wear lighter or less gear. Warm and cool also are relative, however. If you are walking, which generates less heat than running, you are probably cool. When I was training hard, I tended to be warmer, as my pace, even from the beginning of the run, was quicker.

Buy in the right season. For the best selection, shop in late September or early October for fall and winter wear, and in April or May for summer wear. You'll not only have more to choose from, but you'll save time, since you won't have to go from store to store looking for out-of-stock items. Of course, this also depends on geography. People who live in the South can find good summer wear all year long.

Shop when the stores are least crowded. This will increase your chances of getting the most attentive sales help. If possible, do your buying right when the store opens or between 2:00 and 5:00 P.M. on a weekday. Weekdays during lunch hour and Saturdays are the busiest times. Sundays can be either busy or quiet. If you're considering a borderline time, it might be a good idea to call the store and inquire.

Consider mail order. This is especially good if you know exactly what gear you need. These specialty services are fairly sophisticated and usually have well-trained staff. Look for advertisements with toll-free phone numbers in the back of sports specialty magazines.

Do your homework. Read sports magazines for reviews of the latest seasonal gear and how to select and buy it. Bring the reviews into the store with you. But don't take this information as gospel; use it as a guide. You have to try things on to see what fits.

Hot-Weather and Indoor Gear

To exercise outdoors in hot weather or indoors at any time, wear shorts and singlets (sleeveless tops) or T-shirts made of one of the new performance fabrics, such as Supplex, a soft nylon. Shirts with sleeves offer added sun protection. Shorts run the gamut from skimpy to baggy. When I was competing on the track in Europe, all the women wore what looked like bikini bottoms. I ran my first marathon in these. I later heard that people joked that I was running in my underwear. Running shorts, usually split on the sides, have been the standard for years, but the newest trend for runners and walkers are larger, baggier shorts, modeled after soccer or volleyball shorts. These shorts are more versatile for cross-training and give more coverage than the typical running shorts.

Running in Norway and Europe, I never had to worry about sun exposure. Now that I spend time in Florida, I wear sports sunglasses (the wraparound type for maximum eye protection) and a visor. Although sports sunglasses can be expensive, I think it pays to invest in them, not only for protection but also for comfort. They are slip resistant and weigh much less than standard sunglasses.

Cold-Weather Gear

The way some people dress for cold-weather exercise never ceases to amaze me. I've seen people running in shorts in 22°F weather and even remember one woman who wore a running bra and shorts when the temperature was below freezing. These days, you don't have to sacrifice comfort or style to exercise in cold-weather gear.

In terms of clothing, I think the most radical change has come in this type of gear. Twenty years ago, if it was cold, we just wore more clothes, usually sweat-absorbing cotton. They weren't scientifically designed. Although you can probably get away with a T-shirt and shorts outdoors in summer or indoors at other times of the year, I believe that you benefit from wearing state-of-the-art gear in winter.

When selecting outdoor exercise gear, it is important to know whether you want gear for cool weather or cold weather. That's because this clothing ranges from microfiber to polar fleece (for the most extreme conditions). "There is an enormous number of these products," Jones says. He notes that sales help is very important when purchasing winter clothing. I couldn't agree more. Buying and wearing what's appropriate will prevent poor choices or problems. I don't like to be in a situation where I haven't layered my gear properly. I particularly don't like tying extra clothing around my waist after I've warmed up.

Keep in mind that wearing several mid- to lightweight layers is better than wearing two heavy layers. Clothing varying in weight and construction offers many layering possibilities. If it is a very cold day, like those during a Norwegian winter, choose thermal clothing made of heavy fleece, which will wick perspiration away from your body, as opposed to several layers of cotton.

Leg wear also has changed radically over the years. One of the greatest advances has been nylon-spandex tights. I wear all different thicknesses and styles of these tights. Jones says that less form-fitting pants, called tracksters, are now more popular than tights. Pants and tops are usually sold separately.

The greatest advance in winter gear may be in what you *don't* have to buy. "There is almost no reason to purchase a bulky jacket unless you are exercising in extreme conditions," Jones says. "With the advances in fiber technology, there are jackets that are very lightweight, that are windproof and/or highly water resistant."

The body's greatest heat loss is from the head and extremities. In terms of head gear, if it's a fairly mild day, a standard baseball cap or cotton hat is fine. If it's colder, you're better off with the newer fabrics, available in a wide range of styles. The same is true for gloves and mittens. Below 20°F, I wear either a pair of ski gloves (for serious cold) or two pairs of gloves and/or mittens.

Socks also are made in performance fabrics. In colder weather, I make sure to get socks that come up to my calves, so there is no space between the bottom of my pants and the socks. Also, if the toe seams of the socks feel as if they might cause blisters, I turn the socks inside out so that the seam won't rub against my skin.

For Women Only

An exercise bra is probably the most important, and potentially most problematic, piece of exercise clothing a woman can buy. That's because when it's good, you can forget it's there. But when it's bad, it's all you can feel and think about. Running bras are particularly important, since running is a high-impact sport.

I wish I could say that I am an expert on this subject, but I'm far from it. Before I started running marathons, I was at least well enough endowed to wear a bra. Since there were no running bras back then, I had to tie the straps of a traditional bra together in the back with dental floss to keep them from slipping. When I began doing the heavy mileage associated with marathon training, my breasts became smaller, and I stopped wearing a bra. This is perfectly acceptable (from a medical point of view) for women who are small-breasted.

All types of sports bras are available—even tops with built-in bras (called shimmels). The real challenge in the bra industry has been to create a product that is comfortable and effective for large-breasted women. According to Jones, significant advances have been made in this area. High-tech fabrics have long been used in sports bras, but now athletic underwire bras also are being made for women who need more support.

Be just as thorough when purchasing a bra as when buying running shoes. Find a place with experienced sales help (female, if that is more comfortable for you). Try on the bra; it should be snug but allow you to breathe comfortably. With the bra on, move around: Twist, turn, raise your arms and swing them in a running motion, and jump up and down. Take off the bra and run your fingers over all the seams to make sure they are flat and smooth, with no potential source of irritation. Purchase a new bra as soon as the old one shows signs of wear but before it breaks down (no longer offers support). Sports bras are made of the same high-performance fabrics as other new gear. To help maintain their shape and durability, it's best not to put them in the dryer.

Shopping for Shoes

When I first started running, there were no running shoes, just flimsy sneakers or spikes for track running. Good running shoes didn't come on the market until the mid-1970s.

Over the years, I have worn nearly every type of running shoe, depending on my needs (long-distance training or racing, track training or racing). I pay attention not only to the changing shoe technology but also to the evolution of my feet. Changes in foot size and shape are not uncommon for longtime runners. Since I began my career, my foot has grown one full shoe size and my arch has fallen. Of course, my running and exercise needs, and thus my shoe needs, have changed.

I realize I'm in a better position than most people, since I have unlimited access to shoes. But this is such an important part of your exercise life that it pays to invest the time and money it takes to get the best product. It's not necessary, but it's nice to be able to switch shoes if you can afford to have more than one pair. I like the variety in feeling, and because all shoes wear differently, switching shoes is useful for injury prevention, as different shoes stress and rest different parts of the body.

Tips from the Top

I always seek out and use the latest reflective gear, since I often begin my runs in the early-morning darkness. If you exercise outdoors in the dark (including the semidarkness of dawn or dusk), make yourself visible to drivers. Scores of reflective products are made for this purpose, including reflective vests and self-adhesive strips that you can put on your own clothing, as well as gear that features all-over reflectivity. In the latter case, a material is applied to the garment when it is manufactured. With this material, every move you make is visible (including the swinging of your arms), as opposed to the limited view created by a few reflective pieces. Clearly, the greater your visibility is, the greater your safety. Just make sure to carefully follow the washing instructions on this special reflective gear to maintain its efficiency.

By all means, invest in specialty shoes. If you're a runner, buy running shoes and replace them periodically. Many people come up to me in clinics with vague complaints of aches in the lower body. I always look down at their shoes and inquire about them. Often they say that although they've worn the shoes for several years, they still look (and feel) as good as new. Yikes! I certainly wouldn't tell a person to discard a good pair of shoes, but after the soles have compressed and the support is gone, it is time to buy a new pair.

Depending on your running style and the conditions under which you run, you should change shoes after about 500 miles or six months. Some people get more wear from shoes, some less. Walkers don't generate as much force on their feet, so their shoes generally don't wear out as quickly. If you are in doubt, take your old shoes to the store and try on one new shoe and one old shoe. If the new shoe offers noticeably more support, it's time for a change.

We all have different shoe needs, but because I have no specific foot or running gait problems, I choose shoes based on comfort and cushioning. When I was competing, I tended to wear lighter-weight shoes, but now I don't mind if they are a little heavy. I think the older you get, the more cushioning you need. You just have to be careful not to sacrifice support and stability for a soft, lightweight shoe.

According to Chris Jones, shoes are the most critical part of your workout gear, so take time and care when you shop for them. "Don't assume one pair of shoes is just like the next," Jones points out. "You're not always getting exactly the same shoe, even if it's the same brand." With that in mind, here are some tips to help you find the perfect pair for you.

Never assume that a shoe will fit. Always put shoes on both feet and over socks that you will use for exercise.

Walk or run around. If you can, go outside on the sidewalk and test the shoes, or at least wear them on a hard surface which best duplicates where they will be used. Shoes should feel good right out of the box. They generally don't require breaking in, as they once did.

Make a transition. If you're prone to blisters, try using the removable inner sole from your old shoes in your new ones for a few runs.

Bring in your old shoes. A good salesperson can tell what type of stride you have by looking at your worn shoes. Also, if necessary, let the clerk see you run in three situations: barefoot, in your old shoes, and in your new shoes. This will help the salesperson suggest the right shoes for you.

You can do more than run. Running shoes are fine to wear for some other exercises, such as cycling and walking. But do not wear them for aerobics, basketball, tennis, or other activities with lateral movement.

Seek out a low-pressure salesperson. A good salesperson won't try to talk you into a shoe purchase. In addition, the clerk should be willing to let you take the shoes home and walk around in them for a while.

Buy with confidence. Don't leave the store concerned that the shoes are not right for you. If possible, bring them home or to the gym and try them out on a treadmill. Using a treadmill will keep them clean, as opposed to wearing them on a trial road run. Jones suggests that you carry them to the treadmill and take them off when you're done. "As long as the shoes can be resold, the store should take them back," he says.

Go with your gender. In general, women should wear women's shoes. Their feet are different from men's, and women's shoes are usually best for them. There are some rare exceptions, such as myself. My feet are very broad, and I have a bunion, so I have always worn men's shoes.

Exercise and Health
for Everyone

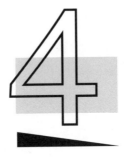

14

Family Fitness
Staying Healthy Together

Family fitness is one of the most crucial topics in the health field—and it's also one of the ultimate pleasures in life. We live in a busy world; we're all under time pressures. But where family is concerned, we must go beyond the usual excuses and find the time and energy to devote to family fitness.

Currently, the state of youth fitness is disastrous. According to the President's Council on Physical Fitness and Sports, nearly half of American youths ages 12 to 21 are not vigorously active on a regular basis. The schools also aren't providing students with adequate exercise. Daily enrollment in physical education classes has dropped from 42 percent to 25 percent among high school students. Most frightening are the health statistics: 40 percent of children from five to eight years old show at least one heart disease risk factor—physical inactivity, obesity, even elevated cholesterol and high blood pressure.

Things are not much better in my native Norway. When I was growing up, all the young people had cross-country skis and used them as often as they could. This is not true today. Downhill skiing and snowboarding are more common, and children are less active. One study of a group of nurses conducted by my former coach, Johan Kaggestad, showed that people in their forties and fifties were in better physical shape than those in their twenties. Kaggestad concluded that the older nurses had better lifestyle habits, which were acquired from their more active childhood days. He also found that a high percentage of young people experienced problems such as headaches and back pain, often caused by inactivity. This trend is found in other Western cultures as well. In 10 European countries and Canada, there has been a steady increase in sedentary activities among preteen and teenage children.

Among the President's Council's findings is the fact that, in general, "social support from family and friends has been consistently and positively related to regular physical activity." Indeed, the United States and, to a lesser degree, other parts of the world experienced a fitness boom in the 1980s. But what happened to the children? It seems that there has been a missing link between adults and children in this area. This must change, which is why I, as well as many experts, stress family fitness.

Meeting the Challenge of Children

Although cultivating physical fitness in children can be a rewarding job, it's not an easy one. It takes a lot of time and attention from parents who are already busy and distracted. When I was growing up, it would have been unreasonable for me to expect my parents to participate in sports activities with me. My father worked very long days, and his job at a pharmaceutical factory—which involved a lot of lifting and moving—was already very physical. When he got home, he was tired. My mother, who worked full-time in a grocery store, also was on her feet all day.

I was lucky, though. I had a network of neighborhood friends who were constantly playing and being active. When I was 12, I joined a sports club. These days, if left to their own devices, children are more likely to pursue a sedentary and unhealthy lifestyle. That's why it often takes active parental interaction to make sure children get the right health and fitness foundation.

Younger children in particular appreciate the presence of their parents and, if possible, their participation with them in sports and games. This active role may need to be tailored as time goes on, especially in the preteen and teen years.

As a child gets older, parents must walk a fine line between being supportive and being overly interested. Sometimes children who are involved in fitness or sports do so only to please their parents. When I see a child who is too serious about sports, I very often see a misguided parent. Also, from an adult perspective, active encouragement may backfire. Parents often come up to me with their children, bragging about their sports accomplishments. I can see the kids getting embarrassed, and I feel embarrassed for them. If you have an athletically talented child, be sensitive to the type of enthusiasm and support they may need.

I also tell parents that each child is different. In my case, my parents weren't initially very interested or involved in my sports activities. I had my peers for company, and I needed to develop my interests myself. By the time I was about 15 and I was much more serious about running, my parents' more active support became important.

Negotiating this arena can be as difficult as finding your way through a field of land mines. We want our children to be active, and if they are talented, we want them to pursue that talent. I suggest that parents look for role models: parents or professionals you admire for doing a good job with child athletes. Also, make sure that the people who are working with your children are able and wise enough to develop each child's ability at a proper, natural pace.

My Own Lessons in Family Fitness

I am not a parent, but I am a full-time aunt. My brothers and I are part of a close-knit family, and I have been very involved in their children's lives.

Fast Fitness

There is no greater reward than sharing the joys of an active, healthy family life. But you don't have to share only sports and other traditional physical activities with your children. A physical life can be anything from dancing to tree climbing. When I was young, dance lessons, which I took for a while, were quite common. My husband started dancing when he was six and went on to become the Norwegian Junior Latin American Dance Champion. An experiment involving folk music was recently conducted among sedentary youths at a Norwegian school. Folk music was played over the public address system during recess, and before long the teens started dancing. It proved to be extremely successful in improving both the teens' attitudes and their physical activity.

My brother Arild has a daughter and a son (Synne, 22, and Espen, 18); my brother Jan has two sons (Geir, 28, and Terje, 25). I am close to all of them, but especially Jan's sons. Although Geir and Terje are now married with children of their own, I was a big part of their lives when they were growing up. When they were young, the boys joined Vidar, my own sports club. They participated in all the club's activities—cross-country skiing in winter, track and field in summer, soccer and other activities at other times of the year. I liked to go to their track meets, and I always asked them about their training. I thought they were having fun; I was happy they were involved.

When Geir was about 13, he got up the courage to ask me to stay away from his sports activities. I was a bit hurt, but I learned that the boys thought we expected them to be champions. They perceived our interest as pressure. Our fault, if there was one, was that we were too interested. Also, maybe if I had not been a world-class athlete, it would have been different.

This experience changed the way I viewed adult involvement with youth sports. It alerted me to the fact that we have to be sensitive to relating to them on their own terms. I don't have all the answers, but we must have done something right, because today my niece and nephews are health and exercise conscious. They know the benefits of being in good shape, and they live an active lifestyle. Your children can, too. Here's what I learned, based on my experience with Geir and Terje and from my years of working with children and youths.

First and foremost, communicate. If you aren't sure what kind of involvement your children want, ask them outright. Early on, begin a dialogue, and continue to communicate as their needs change.

Be aware of what they want. Be careful not to base children's activities or training on your own standards. You're a grown-up. You may think you know what children like, but they often enjoy different aspects of exercise than adults.

Vary their exercise. For your children to find the right activities, they must do several different things at different levels of performance and competition. Because Geir and Terje are three years apart, their skills varied, and we tried to do a little of everything with them.

Start them early. The early school years (beginning in kindergarten) are the time to begin the health and fitness habit. If you start your children young enough, exercise will become a natural part of their lives.

Provide some atmosphere. As vital as it is to vary the sports your children try, it's just as important to expose them to the different environments where physical activity can take place. For instance, we spent a lot of time outdoors, given our enjoyment of the Norwegian forests. But we also did some activities indoors or on a track.

Make a family day out of fitness. Whatever activity you choose, make sure it's something in which the entire family can get involved. It doesn't have to be an obvious sports activity. We used to bike, go walking, or go berry picking. Other athletic activities include climbing trees, throwing stones, and walking on beams or logs. The list is endless, and every activity counts.

Keep it seasonal. Each season brings its own kind of activity. Take advantage of that. In winter, you can go snow hiking or skiing. In summer, focus on water sports. Swimming is great, but don't limit yourself. Water games, deep-water running, or treading water also are useful physical activities.

Be a role model. Where you lead, your children will follow. Let

Should Kids Run?

Running is a good basic sport, but when children are young, they should be doing a variety of activities to develop overall fitness. My advice is not to specialize in a sport before puberty. As a young athlete, I participated in a variety of activities, including shot put, cross-country skiing, and gymnastics. Not only did this allow me to dabble in different sports, but it gave me a good base of strength and flexibility.

them see what exercise you do, and then offer to do it with them.

Look around the neighborhood. What's going on in your community? Is there an open market, street fair, or other event that you can use as an opportunity to walk, be outdoors, and be together? Look in your newspaper for walkathons, bike-a-thons, or fairs that might include games for the kids.

Take exercise to your school or community. Physical fitness often gets overlooked. Help raise teachers' and other parents' awareness. Speak to them about exercise and organize fitness events. If you can pull the wagon together, the burden is easier. Take charge. Be innovative. Try a phone chain to organize a play day or pickup soccer or basketball games. It often doesn't take much to become a fitness leader.

Set a good example. What you eat and when and how you exercise have a powerful influence on your children. If you participate in races, take the children along. Make a day of it, or have them pick you up at the health club and see what you do there.

Keep it fun. Your goal is to get children to participate in activities, not to be a sports coach. Remember, kids won't do it if it isn't fun. I know this from personal experience. As a youth, running at the club was combined with a lot of group activities, from other track-and-field events to overnight camping trips. I would not have continued running if the overall experience had not been fun.

Get educated. Share information with other parents and experts who have developed youth or family fitness activities or programs. You can also do this by contacting organizations such as the President's Council on Physical Fitness and Sports or the Road Runners Club of America.

Being Creative

One challenging part of a child's fitness is the issue of competition. Sometimes competition can be fun, but it also can put a lot of pressure on the child. That's why when my nephews were young, we tried to do activities in which we focused less on competition and more on participation. We played games such as stickball, tennis, and volleyball, but we didn't keep score. We also enjoyed completely noncompetitive activities, such as bike riding and playing hide-and-seek.

Sometimes children express an interest in competition. Competing can be very healthy if it is done on a low-key basis. Following are a few examples of creative competition taken from running games I played with my nephews. We also did these games during cross-country skiing by setting up slalom courses.

Closest, not fastest. This game purposely does not favor the speedster. Each runner runs a loop and records the time. Then the players run the loop again and see who comes closest to matching his or her first time.

Predict a time. In this game, each runner estimates the time it will take him or her to run a specified distance or loop. At the end, you can see who comes closest to the predicted time.

Obstacle course. This is one of my favorites, with lots of variety for kids. When you set up an obstacle course, be sure the obstacles combine skills such as running, jumping, and climbing.

Watching Out for Our Daughters

It always amazes me that in a country so far ahead in so many areas, the United States is so behind in social and athletic equality for girls and women. Today in Scandinavia, we are much better at giving just as much encouragement to girls as to boys.

Young girls face some unique problems when it comes to being active and participating in sports. For instance, whereas boys' bodies change in favor of sports by becoming bigger and stronger, girls become rounder, grow breasts, and often put on weight. I had this problem briefly when I was 14. I came home from a three-week vacation with my brother's family, and the first thing my mother said when she saw me was, "I think I have to put a lock on the refrigerator." Actually, she was very helpful in explaining proper nutrition, and the extra weight soon melted away.

I was lucky to have my mother's support at home, but in general girls' sports were not supported in Norway at that time. Claiming a lack of funds, the Track and Field Federation had no program to support gifted females ages 16 to 19—an important time in a woman's life.

In 1985, I began the Grete Waitz Project, a five-year plan financed by proceeds from the Grete Waitz Run. During those five years, we held training camps for top female runners, who were closely advised and coached. A few of them, now in their twenties, are running pretty well. In fact, three of them made it to the World Championships in 1995.

You don't have to start your own project to foster girls' interests in sports. Here are some suggestions, adapted from material by the Women's Sports Foundation in East Meadow, New York, that you can follow.

Discuss the options. Depending on her size, physical build, speed, and strength, a young female athlete may have several activity options. She may want to talk to coaches or other athletes about their choices and experiences. Make sure you help her to get answers to her questions and to pursue the options that interest her.

Make her activity a family affair. Regardless of the outcome of a contest or competition, the activity is special to your child. It should be something the family shares and enjoys together. You can show your support as a family in a variety of ways. I exercised with my brother. Eventually, he even built a trophy case for me. My parents let me drop piano lessons to pursue running. They also made sure that I had the proper equipment. My father took me to buy my first pair of running shoes.

Show your support. If you cannot attend a contest or game, be sure to indicate your interest and support in other ways. Ask for a full postgame report and learn her teammates' names. My parents knew all the names of my training mates and what sports we played. Ask a lot of questions about the sport. Let her teach you. Become a student of the game or activity. Share books and articles, along with discussions about strategy and coaching. Just be aware of that fine line that I mentioned earlier. Make sure your genuine interest isn't really pressure for her to succeed.

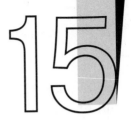

Aging
Growing Older and Sprier

I used to joke that exercise doesn't necessarily help you to live longer, but you *will* die healthier. Despite what science proves or disproves about the effects of exercise on aging, isn't it enough to know that being in shape will help you to live a better life as you age? By being fit, you will be able to do more than your peers. Hiking, playing with your children and grandchildren, biking, and walking are just a few of the many exercise opportunities for fit people, no matter how old they are.

To illustrate this point, consider the consequences if you are not in shape. The more out of shape you are, the more you limit yourself. Daily tasks such as housework, shopping, and walking up stairs become hard work. Many people my mother's age end up feeling lonely and isolated. If my mother weren't in shape, she also would be forced to stay indoors, with only the television for company. In the end, inactive people relinquish the power to care for themselves to doctors and medicine.

It doesn't have to be this way. As you get older, you have a tremendous opportunity to improve your fitness, often much more so than in

171

earlier years. Life is often more settled as you age. Those hectic days of full-time work and child rearing are replaced by retirement and the empty nest. Finding time for exercise becomes easier, as you no longer need to fight the clock to fit it in. I won't say that exercise totally cures the blues that may result from life passages as we age. But if you make it a solid foundation of your life, it can provide relief, comfort, and pleasure. For exercise to serve you well as you age, it is important to get into the habit as early as possible.

My Life as an Aging Exerciser

I am always being asked if my fitness has declined with age and, if so, when the process began. Yes, as I've gotten older, my fitness level has diminished. I can no longer perform as a world-class athlete. Clearly, I am using my running and exercise differently, but the pleasure and benefits that I get from them have not diminished.

When I was performing at a high level, I was aware that my ability began to lessen at a certain point. It's hard to pinpoint exactly when, but I would say it started between ages 34 and 36. It occurred because of my "running age," not necessarily my biological age. After so many years of such intense physical effort, I realized I needed more time to recover. My body didn't heal as quickly when I got injured, and those injuries became more frequent.

I wasn't particularly aware of what was happening at the time. When you are at a relatively young age, you believe you are invincible. You hear about a slowdown, but it doesn't affect your thinking. If I had had a better understanding of this process, I would have handled the last five years of my career very differently. I would have adapted my training and been more patient with myself.

Facing the Future

How do you face the aging process? How do you adapt your exercise? Keep in mind that the effects of aging will inevitably appear. Just

Fitness Facts

As in other Western nations, people in Norway are living longer. In my country, 85 percent of the women and 71 percent of the men reach age 70. Professor Peter F. Hjort, M.D., Ph.D., is a medical professor of geriatrics and an expert on exercise and older people. The following facts come from his book *Physical Activity, Health, and Economy* (Confederation of Sports, 1996).

- Aging is inevitable, but the diseases associated with aging don't have to be. We can protect ourselves with physical exercise.
- Physiologically, older people benefit just as much from exercise as do younger people.
- A very important point for older people: You need very little exercise to achieve beneficial effects. In fact, younger people need more exercise to achieve the same results. These results include better physical fitness and endurance; increased muscle mass and flexibility; better functioning and balance; and increased blood circulation to the brain, which helps improve memory and well-being, while reducing depression.
- Physical activity reduces the risk of death, especially as a result of heart and cardiovascular problems. Those who have heart and cardiovascular disease or weakness may live longer if they exercise.
- Exercise reduces the tendency to get sick. In addition to lowering the incidence of heart and cardiovascular disease, it also reduces diabetes, osteoporosis, and some types of cancer (colon, prostate, and possibly breast cancer).
- Research has shown that rehabilitation after sickness (especially heart attacks) or injury is easier and quicker with patients who are used to being physically active and who were in shape before they got sick.
- Running an average of 25 miles per week over the course of several years does not give people chronic injuries as they get older. The opposite is true. As runners age, they are fitter and have fewer visits to the doctor's office than nonrunners.

as I didn't listen to my body, a lot of people ignore the signs and force themselves to overtrain until they break down. I meet people all the time who tell me that they can't do what they used to, but they won't accept this situation and try to learn from it.

When you feel the effects of aging in your exercise, don't get frustrated or depressed. There's nothing wrong with you; it's just part of life. This realization hits those of us who excel in sports a lot harder, as we have tangible, objective proof that we are getting older: our times on the race clock.

I look at it this way: The years go by whether I want them to or not. I don't worry about what I can't control. It's like fretting about the weather before a race. I can't control it, no matter how much I pray or watch the Weather Channel. Maybe that's why I've won marathons in 80°F and 20°F weather. I don't spend precious energy where I shouldn't.

Peaking Beyond 40

My brother Jan is an example of someone who has benefited from exercise as he has aged. Although his sports participation has been consistent, it has never been his life and his career. Like most people, he has made certain life passages: He grew up, had a family, built a business. Yet through it all, he has artfully adapted his exercise to both his life and his age.

As a teenager, Jan was very active. He began to train seriously at age 17, playing team handball, cross-country skiing, and running. But unlike many young people, he remained active as he grew older. Although you'd expect his peak years to have been between ages 20 and 30, it wasn't practical for him to focus on sports then. His two sons were born, and he was starting his business. The height of Jan's sports training actually came between ages 30 and 40, a time when he could adapt his job to flextime. During that period, he trained for 2 hours a day to compete in cross-country skiing, in which he excelled. Later, he switched his emphasis to running (but still pursued cross-country skiing), because he had the opportunity to train seriously with me. This culminated in his 2:29 marathon best in London in 1983.

Jan says he began to feel his age right after he turned 40. He realized he was more fatigued the day following a hard workout. And when he did train hard, he needed more time to recover. "From ages 30 to 40, I felt nothing was impossible; I felt I could do everything," he says. "After 40, I didn't have that invincible attitude. I began to evaluate, be more conservative, listen to my body more." By age 50, Jan had reduced his training load from daily workouts to exercising three or four times a week, while still holding down a physically demanding job.

How does he compare his past training to the exercise he does these days? "The main difference is that everything takes longer—to warm up, to get loose. Not only is the running slower, but I can't count the first 10 minutes at all. I'm just getting myself started."

Jan also is more conscious of his diet. "At 30, I ate all the time, and I could eat anything. Now I gain weight more easily, so I make sure to eat healthy. I'm not a fanatic, but I keep track." He passes up margarine and butter, sauces, typical fast food, and sweets.

Aging doesn't distress Jan. He realizes that he can still stay in shape. What motivates him now is personal reward—traveling to races in Hawaii or New York City, for instance, where he not only makes use of his training but also socializes with a group of friends. And he still has goals. I think it's pretty great that my 53-year-old brother, a grandfather of three, intends to run sub-3-hour marathons as long as he can. When those days are over, he says he will shift his goal to running sub-3:15 marathons.

Age 65—And Just Getting Started

My mother, Reidun Andersen, began exercising at age 65. What took her so long? Like those to whom this book is directed, she was busy. "I was working long days, rearing three children, and running the ship," she says. "I didn't even think of exercising. Very few of us did in those days. Besides, I got more than enough exercise just doing what I did." But she does regret not starting earlier.

By the mid-1980s, when the Grete Waitz Run for women was well established, I said to my mom, "Why not try to do it?" She said, "No, no, I can't." Every year, though, she loyally watched. In 1989, without telling any of us, she walked the course, just to see what it was like.

"Next year you'll be there with a number on your chest," I told her—a command from daughter to mother.

That was the beginning of her exercise habit. She began running and walking regularly. When her hip started giving her problems several years ago, she took up swimming to supplement her walking, but she still likes walking best. "I like to get out in the fresh air. I sleep better, and I get a nice feeling of fatigue. I would rather be tired from exercising than be tired from doing nothing," she says.

My mom stresses the importance of having friends to exercise with. This is not only fun but also time-efficient. You can socialize and exercise at once. In fact, Mom now has a hard time exercising alone—ever since she found a path in the neighborhood where she met some walking mates.

My mom watches her diet, too. Unlike many older people who live alone, she cooks for herself and eats properly. She sets aside time to make her own meals and has made some small adjustments in diet, such as reducing fats, to safeguard her health.

My mother's goal is to remain active for as long as she can. I applaud her efforts, especially when I see the many people her age who can't do half of what she does.

Making It to the Masters

Masters competition in many sports has become increasingly popular. Masters in some sports are age 35 and up and are usually divided into 5- or 10-year age categories. In running, masters begins at age 40. Since I retired at age 38, people often ask if I ever considered racing as a master. I was never interested. As a competitor, I knew what it was like to have my entire life focused on running. Perhaps if I had not been injured so much after age 35 and hadn't already been running for so many years, the prospect of masters competition would have been more appealing.

When I retired from competition, I decided to give myself two years away and see how I felt at 40. By that time, I was so happy that I didn't see the need to go back. I wanted to get on with my life. I have been able to keep all the good memories and experiences of my running but leave pressure, risks, and twice-daily workouts behind.

Even though I'm not into masters competition, I think that it's great for others. It allows older people to experience competitive sports in conjunction with other life responsibilities. Even if you're a busy exerciser, it's possible to dabble in this competition. Many adults consider masters competition an entirely new endeavor. And because they may be new to the sport, they can experience concrete improvements. This gives them motivation, confidence, and inspiration. You don't have to win or even be competitive to realize the benefits. Just finishing well in your age-group is often affirmation enough.

Wisdom on Aging

Here are some aging facts from sports injury specialist Gerard Hartmann.

- Physical performance measures generally improve rapidly during childhood and reach a maximum between the late teens and age 30.
- Peak muscle strength of men and women is generally achieved between ages 20 and 30. Thereafter, there is a progressive decline in strength. The average male loses 6.6 pounds of muscle with each decade after young adulthood. The rate of loss increases after age 45.
- Between ages 20 and 65, the average person doubles the ratio of fat to muscle.
- Beyond a certain age, we must take a more total view of health, fitness, and performance. We know the various aging facts, but science has proven, and role models show, that the effects of aging can be diminished. You can increase strength and flexibility at any age. You also can change body composition and attain more muscle mass.

Women
Cutting-Edge Findings and Advice

I guess you could say I was a tomboy (we call it "boy/girl" in Norwegian)—and nothing changed that fact, no matter how many dresses and bows my mother tried to make me wear.

I was a physically active, sports-oriented child. (With two older brothers around, that was not surprising.) At first, being a girl posed no obstacles in the sports I played. They were just fun and games. But when I got more serious about track and field, I started to encounter some problems. A girl wasn't supposed to take sports beyond the hobby stage; she was supposed to use her time mainly for schoolwork, piano lessons, gymnastics, or dance. I was happiest as an athlete, so I stayed with sports, and doing so has provided me with many benefits as a woman and a person. I believe that every woman can and should be able to enjoy these benefits.

Sports gave me a core of strength. When I began to excel, sports validated the results of discipline, dedication, and hard work. Participation taught me not to be afraid of setting goals, of reaching for the brass ring. In sports, as in life, nothing is free. I was involved in track and field for years before I achieved good results, but I learned that if you are patient, there is payment down the road. Even when I became a Norwegian National Junior Champion at 16, I knew it would be several years before I could reach my ultimate goal: to make an Olympic or World Championship team.

Being a young female athlete, I had a lot in common with today's busy women. I felt I had to do it all. As the only girl in the family, and with both my parents working, I had certain responsibilities. I had to shop, help cook, and make sure the house was in order. On top of all this, I also had to keep up my grades. And, of course, I had my training. These obligations forced me to be very organized and efficient. That's when I learned how much you can do by developing the skill of careful planning.

Working...and Working Out

Today's typically ambitious woman epitomizes the life of the busy exerciser. She's trying to do it all, while sacrificing little or nothing. I think women are still carrying the weight of the old traditions and expectations: taking care of the house and the children and combining that with pursuing their own careers. And when they can't do it all, they tend to be hard on themselves. They feel a guilt that men usually don't share.

Sports helped me to handle this type of pressure and guilt. As an athlete, I gained the self-confidence I needed to pursue my goals as a person—not just as a woman. But because being a female athlete put me outside the norm, I decided that there were no rules governing what a woman should or shouldn't do. For example, it's OK to ask my husband to clean the house and do the laundry. In fact, in terms of housework, he's better at it than I am.

In addition to my own experience, I have observed the experiences of thousands of women, including some of the participants in the Grete Waitz Run. They range in age from 12 to 93, and they come from all walks of life. But despite their differences, most of them don't face the same pressures as women in the United States. Life is calmer in Norway. We have a shorter workday (8:30 A.M. to 3:00 or 4:00 P.M., with half an hour for lunch), and there is more leisure time.

I have met many fast-track women in the United States, particularly those in the Chase Corporate Challenge. They don't have everything, but they have an awful lot, and they have created it for themselves. In addition to full-time work, many have children, and some are training to run a marathon. "How do you do it?" I ask incredulously. They tell me how they manage to make time for everything. They like running. It gives them the strength to manage a busy schedule. Just as running helped teach me to order my life, it has helped them to realize that by careful planning and willpower, they can set and maintain their priorities. I admire these women greatly.

Get Going with Grete

What's a busy woman to do?

Take up running or walking. Both are great activities for busy people. What's more, women with no sports background may feel more comfortable doing these low-skill, noncompetitive activities.

Experiment. Exercise and work simultaneously. Get something useful done around the house. Chores can be very physical (they're free exercise), as is any task that requires lifting or walking or causes you to huff and puff.

Find friends. Friends help motivate you and help you to enjoy your exercise. You also can save time by socializing and exercising with friends. The women's running pioneer Nina Kuscsik once said that her early running days with friends replaced the typical coffee klatch. These days, you can spot groups of women exercising everywhere, such as the ones I saw running with matching T-shirts that read "Fast and 40."

Set goals. More than half of the 45,000 women in the annual Grete Waitz Run return to do it again. Many of them train in groups. Having a common goal has helped them stick with their exercise.

Building a Support System

In emphasizing how important exercise is for busy women, I can only relate how running affects my life. It relieves stress and gives me more energy. It grounds me with a general feeling of accomplishment and well-being. Many women say that exercise makes them aware of their bodies in unique and different ways. They feel new muscle sore-

A Woman's Benefits

Here are some physiological benefits for women who exercise, courtesy of *The Body Wise Woman* by Melpomene Institute in Minneapolis, which researches women's health and exercise issues.

↳ **General benefits.** Physical activity can improve cardiovascular fitness, control weight, control mild hypertension, improve posture and appearance, and improve functional and motor abilities. It can increase psychological well-being and lower anxiety levels. Another benefit of physical activity may be lighter menstrual periods. Some women also report relief from menstrual cramping.

↳ **PMS.** Increased blood circulation can decrease bloating and fluid buildup. Beta-endorphins released during physical activity can have a calming effect. Physical activity can enhance relaxation by relieving muscular tension and lessening joint pain. Exercise also increases the effectiveness of insulin, which stabilizes blood sugar levels and can decrease food cravings.

↳ **Menopause.** Physical activity can strengthen bones, tone muscles, and improve circulation, digestion, and elimination. It also can help maintain an appropriate weight and reduce stress.

↳ **Pregnancy.** Women who exercise during pregnancy tend to gain less weight than women who don't. Many women report less back pain and less constipation if they remain active during pregnancy.

ness but also new muscle strength. Exercise enhances their self-esteem.

Exercise also is a great social bond. Very often women who work out have mates and friends who exercise with them. I know this firsthand. If not for my running, I wouldn't be married to Jack; I wouldn't even have met him. For the length of my career, he was at various times my coach, training partner, and support system. Without Jack, I could never have withstood the pressures of my career. And when I succeeded, we shared the joy.

Finding and cultivating a support system is essential, whether it's sharing responsibilities with co-workers or sharing with family members on the home front. A busy woman who exercises is dependent on her family not just for household help but also for emotional support. The family needs to have a positive attitude toward her. And if the house doesn't run as smoothly because her time is divided, the family shouldn't make it an issue.

Coping with Cycles

Much has been written on the physical benefits of exercise for women, but perhaps not as much on the physical issues a woman has to deal with when she exercises. For instance, although I have won competitions during every phase of my menstrual cycle, it can be difficult to motivate yourself during this monthly event. In my serious running days, I always tried to schedule my harder workouts and races around those few difficult days before my period. In general, however, you can benefit from working out on those days. Research shows that being active helps you to deal with the physical discomfort, mood swings, and depression associated with the menstrual cycle.

As we age, our bodies change, and women are particularly sensitive to those changes. Whereas my period used to cause me little discomfort, in the past few years I have had a major mental battle with premenstrual syndrome (PMS). When it hits, I want to sit and do nothing. Sometimes I get very depressed. But once I get going in my exercise, although I may be a little heavy-legged, I feel much better. Getting motivated may be tough, but I know that exercise will relieve the blues and the lethargy.

Start Early

The earlier young women exercise, the better. Here are two ways physical activity can benefit girls, as adapted from material from the Women's Sports Foundation in East Meadow, New York.

↪ One to 3 hours of exercise a week over a woman's reproductive life can bring a 20 to 30 percent reduction in the risk of breast cancer. Four or more hours of exercise a week can reduce the risk by almost 60 percent.

↪ Research suggests that girls who participate in sports are more likely to experience academic success and graduate from high school.

Pregnancy and Menopause

Several natural, but life-altering, situations add to the stress women feel. Although events such as pregnancy and menopause are part of life, there are conflicting opinions about how active women should deal with them.

Pregnancy is a time when listening to your body is perhaps more important than at any other time. Experts confirm the benefits of fit women staying active during pregnancy. But although basic medical guidelines are useful, they can't predict how each pregnant woman will react to exercise. I've designed fitness programs for some of the pregnant runners in the Grete Waitz Project. In terms of running, I never tell a pregnant woman how much to do or for how long. Many women have told me there's a point at which running (and probably fitness walking) feels uncomfortable. As an alternative, I prescribe deep-water running for pregnant athletes. Cross-training—resistance training, riding a stationary bike, or doing some other activity—also can be beneficial.

Some women feel the need to keep up their exercise until their due date, then resume very shortly afterward. I know that it is supposedly safe to exercise this way, but I recommend taking your time. Remember the lifestyle balance I have stressed throughout this book. Pregnancy is a period of discovery, both emotionally and physically. If you're really motivated, your exercise will be there for you when your body is ready. In the meantime, concentrate on taking care of yourself and your newborn.

I've also known women who have lost the motivation to exercise during pregnancy and who aren't inclined to resume working out afterward. I know that having a baby changes a person's priorities, and although the will to work out has to come from within, eventually resuming your exercise routine will benefit both you and your family in the long run.

I haven't reached menopause yet, but I am following the developments in hormone replacement therapy research and the effects of exercise on the mind and body during this time of life. I have taken hormones in the past to bring on my menstrual cycle, which was absent for several years during my competitive career. I know that women are sharply divided on the issue of hormone replacement therapy, but based on what we know today, I believe that I will take hormones when I reach menopause. We all must stay informed on this important topic so that we can each make a knowledgeable decision at that time. One thing is certain: Being physically active and in good shape will help every woman to handle menopause better, both physically and emotionally.

The Psychological Connection

Another aspect of every woman's life is the relationship between exercise, or lack of it, and body image. It is easy for me to tell women to disassociate their exercise from their looks—to accept their bodies as they are. But that advice has little impact in light of the constant barrage of social messages that tell us otherwise.

When I say that participating in sports has taught me a lot, I include the self-knowledge it has given me. I know my strengths and my limitations. I'm good at sports, and I had a wonderfully successful career. But I accept that I can't be good in every area. I can't cook or play the piano very well. I'm not very creative or very adventurous. Just as I can't do it all, when it comes to appearance, I can't have it all. I've got a great body for running, but I'll never model a swimsuit. I have a good sense of humor about myself. To quote a well-known Norwegian comedienne (and friend), I am "the walking asparagus."

It would be insane to say that I'm not grateful for what my body has been able to do. But if I had a "real figure," would I like myself better? I don't know. Life is more than a perfect body. In fact, women who are desperate to lose weight often still are not happy after having done so. Then they have to find the real cause of their unhappiness. For both women and men, exercise is not only the best way to create a healthy body—which I say is the only "perfect body"—but also a great way to learn to accept the way we look and to celebrate ourselves.

17

Nutrition
Fueling for Fitness

We have an expression in Norwegian: "Your food is your medicine." What you eat is what keeps you well and, together with exercise, what keeps you healthy. Eating also is a pleasure, or should be. But I believe that the biggest hurdle to making eating both healthful and pleasurable is obsessing about it. This often results in fad diets, poor nutrition, and the distraction that comes from experimenting with the latest quick fix or new food philosophy.

In Norway, people are not generally obsessed with nutrition. Those in my generation, at least, stick to a basic diet, which is very healthy. Because most of what we eat is native to our country, Norwegian food is fresh, and the typical diet is simple and unprocessed. Most Norwegian dishes are basic and unadorned—and very easy to prepare. In this regard, we are lucky. For us, having a good diet is easy. Like other Europeans, Norwegians shop daily, which means buying fresh. Even when I am in the United States, I shop daily, although many people remark about my frequent visits to the supermarket.

The best way for busy, health-conscious people to have a good diet is to keep it simple and consistent. It also helps to have a thorough understanding of how to get the most from the foods you choose. By using the Norwegian diet as a model, this chapter will help you do exactly that. Along with the foods I have eaten and enjoyed my entire life, I suggest other food choices that have become available more recently.

People always ask me what I ate when I was running competitively. They like to believe there's a special food that's best for athletes. But when it comes to training, there is no magic food or diet. I have always eaten the same diet, although I ate more food when I was running more than 100 miles a week. I always had a good nutritional foundation, which I believe contributed greatly to my athletic success and overall health. My motto is: If it's healthy for an athlete, it must be healthy for the average person.

Eating Like a Norwegian

In Norway, we are fortunate to have an abundance of fruits and vegetables, as well as whole-grain products such as inexpensive fresh bread. We also have a good selection of dairy products such as milk and cheese. My favorite is *gjitost*, a sweet-flavored brown goat cheese that is high in iron. It is sold in the United States under the name Ski Queen. The other Norwegian cheese that is readily available in the United States is Jarlsberg.

Norwegians eat a lot of fish. Whereas chicken is a luxury (a small, roasted supermarket chicken costs about $10), fish is reasonably priced. Norwegians eat some meat, but I have never been a fan of red meat because I don't like the taste or the texture. If you eat meat, look for lean cuts and don't overdo it. Eat the recommended serving—about the size of a pack of cards.

My diet consists of three basic meals a day.

Breakfast. I'm a firm believer in breakfast, a meal widely acknowledged as the most important of the day. Breakfast and my morning workout go together. I never schedule anything before this ritual. If you exercise in the early morning, you should make a postexercise meal part of the plan. It is important to consume fluids and carbohydrates after exercising to refuel the muscles.

I enjoy fairly traditional fare (oatmeal, whole-grain cereal with yogurt, or thick-sliced bread with cheese or jam). Norwegians eat a cereal called muesli, versions of which are also sold in the United States. You can make your own muesli by combining raw oats, dried fruits, and nuts. If you absolutely don't have time to eat breakfast at home, pack it with you. I carry a bagel or banana and purchase a drink. Items you will never see at a Norwegian breakfast include doughnuts, muffins, and Danish. Muffins are not a good choice unless you purchase or bake a nutritious, low-fat variety. If you bake low-fat muffins, freeze them and pop one in your bag before you leave the house.

Lunch. For lunch, if I am home, I make soup or a baked potato with cottage cheese or plain yogurt and a vegetable salt or herb salt. If I'm out on the road, I take a *matpakke*, an open-faced sandwich on thick-sliced bread. The matpakke is a Norwegian institution. Rich or poor, most Norwegians bring these sandwiches, wrapped in white butcher paper, to work or school. We sometimes eat them for supper as well.

When I use the term *sandwich*, I mean it as bread with a little filling, not the other way around, which is often the way I see sandwiches made. A good sandwich is not loaded with filling (vegetables are the exception). The bread in Norway is sliced at least ½ inch thick and is often topped with a small amount of fish, turkey, liverwurst, or cheese (I always use a cheese slicer so that the slices are thin), or hard-boiled eggs (eggs are an important part of the Norwegian diet). On top of the protein layer, we put vegetable toppings: tomatoes, cucumbers, lettuce, pickles, or cooked beets. A traditional sweet variation is strawberry jam topped with banana slices. Toppings are limited only by your imagination. Try grilled vegetables, apple slices, tofu salad (like egg salad), or leftover meatloaf.

My matpakke habit means I am never without a substantial and healthful meal. Although it is not as easy to duplicate these sandwiches outside of Norway (I rely on my mom for homemade bread), any pack-along meal makes it easy for me to carry a healthy lunch with me.

Dinner. My dinner is simple—often salad, rice, or a baked potato. Sometimes, I'll make an omelet or have a small piece of chicken, turkey, or fish. I flavor all my food with a combination of seasonings and herbal salt found in the grocery store.

I have fond childhood memories of my mother's cooking, and I look forward to it every time I go back to Norway. Here are some of my favorites. All of them are nutritious and easy to make.

Mom's Whole-Grain Bread

This bread, which is what my mom supplies me with these days, is a meal in itself. (I have to admit, I don't bake.) Not only is it nutritious and filling, it is low-fat and low-salt. But most of all, it is delicious! In Norway, the open-faced sandwiches we make with bread such as this are a staple. This bread can be baked without letting it rise a second time, but it will be a bit more dense. This recipe makes 4 loaves.

4	cups nonfat milk
3	cups water
14–15	cups whole-wheat flour
2	teaspoons salt
1¼	cups oatmeal
¾	cup bran
3	tablespoons canola oil
3	packages yeast

In a large saucepan, heat the milk and water to 120°F.

In a very large bowl, combine 12 cups of the flour, the salt, oatmeal, bran, oil, and yeast. Mix thoroughly. Knead in the bowl for 3 to 5 minutes, kneading in 2 to 3 more cups of flour. The dough will be slightly sticky. Cover the bowl with plastic wrap. Let rise for 2½ to 3 hours, or until doubled. Punch down.

Spray 4 (8″ × 4″) loaf pans with no-stick spray. Place one-quarter of the dough in each pan.

Cover and let rise for 1 hour, or until dough has doubled. Bake in a preheated 375°F oven for 50 minutes to 1 hour, or until the bread sounds hollow when tapped on the bottom and is lightly brown on top.

Fish Soufflé

This was a special meal because my mom often made it for dinner on her one day off from the grocery store where she worked. I liked to eat it, but I think I liked it even more because she was home and life was more relaxed.

2   tablespoons light margarine
2   tablespoons flour
1   cup low-fat milk
4   eggs, well-beaten
1   pound cod fillet (cut into 1″ cubes)
    Salt and pepper to taste
2   tablespoons bread crumbs

Preheat oven to 350°F. In a medium saucepan, melt the margarine over low heat. Stir in the flour. Gradually add the milk, stirring constantly. Cook until thickened. Stir a little of the sauce into the eggs and then stir the egg mixture into the sauce. Stir in the fish, and salt and pepper to taste.

Spray a 1-quart round casserole or soufflé dish with no-stick spray. Pour in the fish mixture. Sprinkle with the bread crumbs. Bake in the middle of the oven for 45 minutes, or until a knife inserted in the center comes out clean and the top turns golden.

Spinach Soup

This was always my brother Arild's favorite. He would request it on his birthday, and if there was any left over, it belonged to him.

2   tablespoons butter
2   tablespoons flour
    About 1¼ cups water
1¼ cups milk
½   teaspoon dried dill
1   teaspoon lemon juice
1–2 bouillon cubes, chicken or vegetable
1   box (10 ounces) thawed frozen spinach

Warm the butter in a pot. Add the flour, 1¼ cups water, and milk. Add more water if the soup is too thick. Add the dill, lemon juice, bouillon cubes, and spinach. Warm and serve.

Grete's Own Two-Step Tomato-Vegetable Soup

Not that I'm much of a cook, but I do take some pride in having invented this recipe myself, after spending time in the United States and discovering V-8 Juice.

1	can (12 ounces) tomato juice or V-8
¼	pound cooked shrimp, fish pieces, fishballs, or chicken
1	cup frozen or fresh vegetables, such as cauliflower, broccoli, leeks, or squash
1	clove minced garlic
1	teaspoon chopped parsley
	Dash of hot-pepper sauce

Combine the juice, seafood or chicken, vegetables, garlic, parsley, and hot-pepper sauce. Cook over medium heat until the vegetables are soft.

Maximizing Mealtime

In addition to making eating easy, it is important for busy people to make what they eat count. A typical busy person's fare—fast food or precooked supermarket or restaurant food—can compromise good nutrition if you don't know how to make optimum choices. You need not sacrifice quality for convenience; you can have them both.

The same goes for what you choose to cook. Those pressed for time are not inclined to do much shopping and cooking. I am by no means a cook, but I know how to stock a healthy kitchen. And because I move around a lot, I know how to do it simply and efficiently. Since I shop daily, I don't make regular use of my freezer. But if shopping in bulk is more practical for you, use your freezer for nearly everything, including blanched fresh vegetables, some dairy products, and individual meal portions. Following is some advice to help you get the most out of your meals.

Stock your staples. In my kitchen, I always keep a supply of staples from which I can make any of my three daily meals. These include rice (if you use brown rice, refrigerate it; the bran in brown rice contains oil, which can turn rancid), potatoes, bread (which I store in the freezer), frozen vegetables, Scandinavian crispbread (crackers), rice cakes, canned tuna, and vegetable juices such as V-8 and tomato juice.

Breakfast in a Blender

Want a healthy, quick breakfast, but you're not in the mood to eat? Try a yogurt drink. In a blender, combine plain low-fat or nonfat yogurt, a banana or other fresh fruit (optional), orange juice (fortified with calcium for women), and wheat germ (optional). Or create your own combinations of ingredients.

Be particular with pasta. I have never liked pasta, but I know it is a favorite. If you use it, try to eat whole-wheat or buckwheat pasta, or at least combine whole-wheat and white pasta. To maximize the nutrients in pasta, don't rinse it after cooking. Buy pasta in cardboard containers; pasta in clear packaging can lose 30 percent of its riboflavin in just one week's time.

Load up on perishables. My basic perishable items include cottage cheese, hard cheese, sliced turkey, eggs, fruit, salad makings, and frozen vegetables.

Eat heart-friendly fish. Fish is as Norwegian as burgers and fries are American. It is low-fat, easy to digest, and contains everything from omega-3 fatty acids (which have been shown to reduce the risk of heart attack and perhaps stroke) to high amounts of calcium (from the bones in canned salmon and sardines).

In Norway, we have many varieties of fish (it's our main export) and many uses for it. Since I'm not a great cook, I don't trust myself in the kitchen with a good piece of fish. But when I go out, I always turn to the seafood section of the menu. Fish is a good choice for busy people because it doesn't take long to cook. You also can use leftover fish in soups, salads, and sandwiches.

Shop shrewdly. It pays to learn to shop smart. Occasionally, set aside some time to study the supermarket aisles. Read the labels and see what various foods contain. That's what I began to do when I first got interested in nutrition. Take note of what's new and check to see if

Breaking Taboos

People are told to shun salt, but if you're active, you need not be overly concerned about salt (unless you have a medical condition, such as high blood pressure). Active people can use the salt, especially after heavy perspiration.

Eggs also have gotten a bad rap, although a few aren't bad for you. If you are concerned about cholesterol, you can remove some or all of the egg yolks or use an egg substitute.

it measures up to the advertising claims. Buy foods that are nutrient dense—that is, the ones that pack the most nutrition for their size and calorie content. Buy vegetables and fruits in season, when they are least expensive and most nutritious.

Choose for convenience. Not all convenience foods are less nutritious than homemade foods. Some ready-made foods available at Norwegian supermarkets are prepared in kitchens right on the premises. Salad mixes also are a good choice, as they retain their vitamin content despite being prewashed and precut. (That's because the breathable plastic bags they come in are specially designed to keep vegetables fresh.) Salad bars are a great source of fresh vegetables for soups or stirfries.

Embrace the dark side. When you're choosing vegetables, think color: the darker the green, the healthier the vegetable. Dark green vegetables such as spinach, kale, and broccoli are far more nutritious than paler green vegetables such as iceberg lettuce, cucumbers, and alfalfa sprouts. Dark orange produce such as sweet potatoes, carrots, and pumpkins also are high in nutrients. Bananas, apricots, kiwi fruit, papayas, mangoes, oranges, and cantaloupe have it made over green grapes, apples, and plums.

Keep your veggies vital. To keep nutrition content at its highest, wash and cut fruits and vegetables right before cooking or eating, and eat them within a couple of days of purchase. Save (or freeze if necessary) any nutrient-rich water from cooking vegetables. You can use it to make gravy or as soup stock.

Find more fiber. Many of the foods I eat—such as oatmeal, Mom's bread, beans, and grains—are high in fiber and fill me up. Because they keep your blood sugar level stable, they stick with you longer.

When I make my husband his matpakke lunch with three thick slices of bread, it lasts him 6 hours, until he comes home for dinner.

Even if you eat low-calorie, low-fat frozen dinners, you can make them heartier by adding fiber. Serve them with a salad, whole-grain bread, or other additions to make a complete meal. (They're often low-calorie because their portions are so small.) If you like the ease of boiling pasta or microwaving potatoes, try some healthy variations on the standard sauces and toppings, such as thick lentil or bean soup, which will add fiber and flavor.

Try new toppings. There are all sorts of ways to sneak healthy food into your meals, especially with toppings. You can make a great one by pureeing some cottage cheese in the blender with spices. Or puree cooked vegetables (add a little broth if necessary) and use them as sauces or spreads. Use kidney, garbanzo, or other beans on salads or in other dishes. Wheat germ is a great source of vitamin B$_6$, protein, and vitamin E. Sprinkle it on yogurt or cereal or use it in place of bread crumbs, in scrambled eggs or pancake batter, or in baked goods. Add iron-rich raisins, prunes, or other dried fruit to cereal or to meat or vegetable dishes. You can plump dried fruit by cooking it in water. Use this fruit compote over yogurt or as a dessert.

Go lean on your meat. If you use ground beef in your recipes, brown it and drain the fat. To lower the fat content even further, place cooked meat in a colander and rinse it with warm water. Consider switching to ground turkey, ground soy, or tofu. Combine your ground beef with these meat substitutes or other additions such as mashed beans, pureed vegetables, grated vegetables, or grains. This works well for casseroles, meat loaf, or chili.

Freeze the fruit. For fast, healthy desserts, keep fruit chunks in the freezer. Eat them as is or put them in the blender (with a bit of juice if needed) to make a fruit shake. You can also use them to make a topping for frozen yogurt or low-fat cake. In the summer, I freeze orange juice (calcium fortified) to make pops, and in the past I've frozen flavored yogurt for a healthy ice cream–like treat.

Make cooking fun. When you're tired or pressed for time, you may be more inclined to eat fast food or make less healthy choices. That's why it's important to make the time to prepare good meals. Meal preparation may be more pleasurable if you set aside some time to make a week's worth of meals (or main courses) at once and then freeze them. You can even make it a family affair—maybe on a weekend—and let the children take part. This also is a good way to send a positive message about family fitness.

Eating Out

In Norway, we don't have widespread take-out food, except pizza. In addition, people generally don't eat out in restaurants (it's very expensive) unless it's a special occasion. But because I travel so much, I do eat out often. And because I enjoy simple, healthy food, I have learned how to pick and choose in any restaurant. Here's how you can enjoy eating out while still eating healthy.

Make a change. Fortunately, most restaurants now have healthy choices on the menu. But I am never shy about asking the kitchen to adapt my order—to change french fries to a baked potato, put salad dressing on the side, or put plain lemon juice or vinegar on my fish instead of sauce.

Beware of big portions. Many restaurants tend to serve large portions—or at least too much of the entrée. Either share an entrée or ask for a doggy bag to bring half home. Most restaurants are happy to accommodate your request.

Avoid fat friendships. Lone diners consume less than those eating with others. I'm not saying that you should eat by yourself, but be careful. Socializing over a meal with friends or family is great, but you are likely to eat more. Eating out with health-conscious people, however, makes you more inclined to eat healthier, too.

Select the salad. If you're eating out, especially at a typical fast-food restaurant, a salad can be a smart choice. But don't think "salad" automatically means "healthy." Watch for the cheese or meat topping, and beware of tuna or chicken salad made with mayonnaise. Also, make sure to ask for low-fat or nonfat dressing.

Be smart with sandwiches. Don't order chicken or fish sandwiches in a fast-food restaurant unless they are grilled or broiled. Hold all special sauces or extra cheese. And if you're eating a breakfast sandwich, skip the ones that are made with biscuits or croissants: Half of their calories come from fat.

Practice pizza prudence. Pizza is a favorite food, but choose the more "gourmet" varieties, which tend to have less cheese. Get pizzas topped with vegetables—not pepperoni or sausage, which are dripping with fat. Hold some of the cheese. Finally, blot the oil on top with napkins.

Healthful Ethnic Foods

Although I am not a fan of ethnic foods, I know they are popular among restaurantgoers. Here are some tips on how to eat healthier at ethnic restaurants.

- **Italian.** Stay away from casseroles such as lasagna or other dishes with cheese fillings.
- **Chinese.** Ask for food to be steamed, or request that your stir-fried dishes be made with broth, not oil. Go heavier on the vegetables and rice, and choose seafood or chicken over beef or pork.
- **Mexican.** Skip the chips given as appetizers, or ask for steamed tortillas instead, which you can dip in salsa (but watch out for the high-calorie guacamole). Order more traditional Mexican dishes, which rely less on cheese, sour cream, and other fatty additions than the dishes served in typical Mexican-American restaurants.

Go ahead—indulge yourself. Making healthy choices when you eat out is important, but you can overdo it. If going out is a rare treat and you want to indulge yourself, go ahead and do it. You can always compensate by eating less the rest of the day or the next day.

Drinking and Eating

What you drink and when you drink it are just as important as what and when you eat. I learned the importance of hydration the hard way—by having several bad experiences with dehydration in hot-weather races.

Exercisers need to make sure that they get enough fluids before, during, and after working out. In addition, if you are properly hydrated, it helps control your appetite. That's why diet experts recommend drinking plenty of fluids before meals and starting meals with clear soups.

Water is always the fluid of choice. Experts say that you should drink at least eight full glasses a day, even when you aren't exercising. Juices are a traditional drink for health-minded people, but they are very high in sugar and calories. If you choose them, water them down. Better yet, try adding a bit of your favorite juice—a spoonful of frozen juice concentrate or a twist of lemon or lime—to plain seltzer or ice water. You can also freeze juice cubes and add them to plain water. With these methods, you get the taste of juice without all the calories and sugar.

Many people like a preworkout cup of coffee or tea—for the caffeine boost, the ritual, or both. I like an occasional cup of coffee or tea or glass of wine. I drink herbal tea for its taste, not necessarily because it is caffeine free, although that is a benefit for those watching their caffeine consumption.

Snacking and Sweets

Snacks are a sensible, useful part of a healthy diet, particularly for busy people. Snacking has a bad reputation, but it isn't snacking that's the problem; it's the snack choices that people often make. Snacking can be especially important for those individuals who are forced to eat on the run or skip meals. Try to keep a stock of healthy snacks on hand, such as pretzels, fruit, and carrot sticks.

If you like sweets, try to eat them sensibly. Depriving yourself may just make you end up bingeing. By eating wholesome, filling foods, however, you may find that you crave sweets less. Try to eat sweets with meals rather than on their own as snacks. Whenever possible, choose fruit-based sweets (cobbler, a baked apple, or raisin, fig, or other fruit cookies) over candy and chocolate. Try to make desserts yourself, cutting back on the sugar and fat. (That's not hard to do, since the high fat content of commercial sweets is used to increase their shelf life.) To lower the fat content and increase the nutrition, try the new baking substitute fruit purees made from apples or prunes, which are available in grocery stores, or make them on your own.

My motto for sweets—Just say no—works for me, but I know it is unrealistic for most people. Sweets are not a prominent part of the Norwegian diet, and they weren't often present when I was growing up. My brother Arild and I would often make a desperate search through the house for treats. Even the box of raisins my mom saved for cooking was not safe. (I remember a time when she reached for the box, and although it looked as if it was intact, it had been emptied via a carefully carved hole in the bottom.) For years, I used to relax between daily workouts with the newspaper and a few caramels—until my teeth became loaded with cavities. Now I eat fruit or crackers and cheese for dessert or a snack.

Making Supplement Sense

Do active people really need vitamin and mineral supplements? It's always best to get your vitamins and minerals from foods, which I believe you can do with a balanced diet. But since so many people don't have an ideal diet, it certainly doesn't hurt to take a multivitamin. Just be careful not to take megadoses or to take vitamins instead of eating a healthy diet. When I was competing, I took calcium, iron, vitamin C, and vitamin B complex. Now, as an active woman, I concentrate more on iron (taken with vitamin C to enhance absorption) and calcium supplements.

If you do take vitamin and mineral supplements, make sure to take them at optimum times and in optimum combinations, since absorption is key. Supplements are best absorbed with food. Calcium and fiber can block absorption of iron. If, for instance, you eat whole-grain cereal with milk for breakfast, don't take your calcium supplement then. I take my iron with vitamin C (or you can drink orange or tomato juice), separate from my breakfast. I take my calcium in the evening, after dinner.

Do sports bars and drinks help you perform better? As far as sports bars go, if you like them, fine. But you can also get the same carbohydrates from a bagel, a banana, or some figs or raisins. As for sports drinks, they do help replenish fluids and nutrients that are lost after a hard workout. They also are useful in summer or if you work out hard inside a gym, where there is less ventilation. Go ahead and drink them if you like the taste, but they are not as effective if you water them down. Conversely, if you are using a powder to make your own, don't make them thicker than directed. They won't do you any more good, and they may be less digestible. You shouldn't need these drinks unless you are training very hard or perspiring very heavily.

The Fat-Free Fallacy

Among my pet peeves in the health and fitness marketplace are the advertisements for, and overflowing supermarket shelves of, fat-free foods. For example, there are between 100 and 150 brands of low-fat or fat-free cookies on the market today, up from about 3 or 4 in the late 1980s. So if everyone is eating these foods, why aren't people getting thinner? In fact, just the opposite is true: People are gaining more weight than ever. That's because they seem to confuse fat-free with calorie-free.

Some fat-free products are useful, but relying on them can backfire. The nutrition experts tell us that if we crave sweets, for instance, we may be better off having a small amount of the real thing than going for a fat-free product, particularly if we eat a large amount. Personally, I would rather eat a small amount of full-fat, flavorful cheese than a larger portion of a reduced-fat or fat-free variety. If you choose foods that are naturally fat-free—such as fruits, vegetables, whole grains, and legumes—and indulge in a small amount of fat, you'll be better off.

As a world-class athlete, I have seen it all: the high-protein diets, the bee pollen craze, carbohydrate loading for long-distance running. I have always shunned the latest fad and stayed with the basics. That's my motto in training, and it's my motto in nutrition as well.

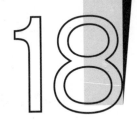

Health from Head to Toe
An Ounce of Prevention, a Pound of Cures

When you're juggling a lot of obligations—work, family, friends, health, and exercise, to name a few—you must be extra careful to maintain balance in your daily life. Of course, your exercise is supposed to keep you healthy, not contribute to your stress. But sometimes the opposite is true, especially in certain situations. Many upsets—including seasonal and weather changes, life and job stresses, and new or increased exercise—can challenge your routine and your health.

I speak from my own experience when I say that you can have a busy life and enjoy your exercise, too. But you have to pay close attention to the fine line you walk. Exercise is about pushing your body, but in stressful situations, you can push too far. When you become overtired or overstressed, you can compromise your immune system. That makes you more vulnerable to colds, flu viruses, and even more serious illnesses. You also are more prone to injury. When you're tired and fatigued, your body's balance, alertness, coordination, and movement are not as good as when you are fresh.

Listening to Your Body

In the past, when I was asked to comment on injuries during my 20-year competitive career, I would come up short. That's because I was rarely injured. In fact, I was hurt seriously—to the point of missing major competitions—only three times, all in the last five years of my career. I consider myself extraordinarily fortunate in this regard.

When I wrote my first book, *World Class,* I had to rely largely on the advice of other experts for information on preventing injuries. I wrote, "Injury prevention is a process of learning to listen to your body communicate with you. Pain is telling you something. Don't shut out the message by ignoring it or trying to cover it up with painkilling medication.... Sometimes, however, I have not been good at listening to my body, because I didn't want to hear what it was telling me. Rest and recuperation, as for many runners, is difficult for me."

Those words just about sum up my advice for injury prevention and most accurately describe not only my own failings but also those I have noticed in many runners and exercisers. I coach several elite athletes who have a difficult time exercising restraint. Every time one of them asks me if she should continue hard training despite some ache or pain, I ask her, "If you were giving advice to someone else in your situation, what would you say?" Like so many of us, these athletes tend to think they are invulnerable, that what applies to others somehow does not apply to them. We are very good at giving advice to other people. If you had a friend who had been working hard or had a sore knee, you'd surely tell that person to cut back on training. But would you do it yourself? Live by the advice you give to others in similar situations. Always remember, when in doubt, back off. And don't fret about losing fitness. Research shows that runners perform better when they are a little undertrained than when they are overtrained. And they don't perform at all when they are injured or sick.

I heard the advice "Listen to your body" thousands of times over my career, but I didn't do it. If there were warning signs, I ignored them. Part of the problem was that in my competitive days, I couldn't rest without feeling guilty. I was on a mission. If my competitors were out training hard, I felt guilty if I wasn't, too. Today I can rest without guilt, and I understand that simply listening to your body isn't enough: You have to heed what it is telling you.

I am a much wiser person now than when I was competing. Much of my knowledge and experience with illness and injury prevention has to do with the combination of aging and having put in many hard miles. When you are 18, you feel invincible. It almost seems that if you broke a leg in the morning, it would be healed by the evening. Recovering from injury and illness doesn't seem so easy when you are 35. Now, in my forties, I notice a big difference in my body. I am less flexible, sorer. It takes more time to recover from hard exercise and longer to heal if I do get injured.

Overcoming Aches and Ailments

People have asked me if a positive mental attitude had anything to do with my being healthy—implying that I just willed away illness and injury. I don't think so. You can't think away a stress fracture. Part of my success, however, was living healthy overall. By that I mean not only a good diet and rest, but also a very stable social and emotional life. I've also always been very organized, being able to get a lot done in a planned and calm manner. My balanced life has helped me to exercise good judgment and common sense—key in minimizing the risk of illness and injury.

For me, injury prevention also means a combination of cross-training, stretching and strengthening exercises, and massage therapy. I discussed stretching and strengthening exercises and cross-training in chapters 8 and 9. The third aspect of my three-pronged approach is massage therapy. As the years go by, I increasingly realize how important massage is. Before I found a good massage therapist, I spent time with plenty of other healers and techniques. When I first encountered hamstring problems, I was treated with laser, ultrasound, and electrical stimulation machines. That was easy for the practitioner, who just hooked me up and moved on, but it didn't really help me. For soft-tissue injuries (any trauma to muscles, tendons, ligaments, or joint capsules), nothing works for me like the hands-on approach of a skilled massage therapist.

Experience also has helped me avoid injuries. I've experienced most of the bodily aches and ailments listed here. From head to toe, wherever they strike, you don't have to let injuries take you out of the race. With a little planning and common sense, you can overcome and even prevent these health problems, too.

Muscle soreness and stiffness. From weekend warriors to marathoners, who among us hasn't experienced sore muscles? I was never stiffer or sorer than after my first marathon. My worst experience, though, was in the 1982 Boston Marathon. I was well ahead of the world record pace (2:23), and 2 minutes ahead of the woman in second, when I hobbled to a stop at 23 miles. My thighs were so beat-up from running downhill and from dehydration that I didn't run a step for 12 days afterward. I had a hard time getting to the other side of the street before the traffic light changed.

Proper training and preparation can prevent most serious soreness, but sometimes you'll be sore after an event or exercise no matter how much you train. When you do feel muscle soreness, here's what you can do.

• Ice and heat. For initial muscle soreness, which is caused by tissue inflammation, ice is the best treatment. Keep a plastic bag with ice cubes on hand, or use a bag of frozen vegetables for the most form-fitting ice pack. But don't just freeze the area. Follow a 10-minutes-on, 10-minutes-off routine. Repeat this time sequence three or four times a day to promote circulation. If you have a plastic ice pack, don't put it directly on the skin, which can cause damage; wrap it in a thin towel. Many people want to sink into a hot bath, but heat is not the proper treatment at first because it increases the inflammation. After 72 hours, you can treat the stiffness that sets in with an Epsom salts bath.

• Anti-inflammatory medication. For muscle aches and soreness as well as for injuries, use an anti-inflammatory medication (usually over-the-counter aspirin or ibuprofen) to reduce swelling and aid healing. I never took this medication for a sports injury unless it was prescribed because it upsets my stomach. If you take an anti-inflammatory drug, take a coated variety, which is easier on the stomach. Or take it with food, especially something that will coat the stomach, such as yogurt. It is best to use this medication only if you absolutely have to.

• Massage. I've had thousands of massages over the years. I've had all different types, from those in which a little oil is rubbed on to those in which you feel as if you've been through a boxing match. Everyone's needs and tastes differ. Although I think a relaxing massage is a wonderful treat that exercisers should allow themselves, I personally like my massage to "hurt good." I want my muscles to be worked, to get out the lactic acid (muscle waste products) and increase the blood circulation. If you want to get a good massage, here's all you need to do.

In addition to reading advertisements or getting a professional referral, find a good massage therapist by word of mouth.

Always ask the therapist whether he or she has worked on athletes. Tell the person what you need or want. If I feel that the pressure of the massage is too light, I tell the therapist to go deeper. Similarly, if it's too hard, I mention that. I once woke up with bruises the day after a massage. That was clearly an overly enthusiastic treatment.

If you are not experienced, be willing to try different types of massage therapists to find out what you like. There are many different styles and philosophies.

Back pain. Most people experience back pain at some point in their lives, whether or not they exercise. Ninety percent of back pain is due to a muscular imbalance. The best treatment and prevention of back pain is stretching and strengthening: doing abdominal and lower back exercises for strength; stretching the hamstrings, quadriceps, and gluteals. I may have had other aches and pains throughout my career, but doing these exercises has helped me avoid back pain.

Chafing. To avoid this problem at crucial times, I never competed in clothes or shoes that I had not worn in training. Check clothing for rough seams. If necessary, wear it inside out to keep the seams from rubbing against your skin. Before exercising, apply petroleum jelly to vulnerable places: around the armpits if you wear a singlet, on the backs of the ankles where shoes can rub, or under bra straps or waistbands.

Sun exposure. Coming from Norway and training in the early morning, I never had a problem with sun exposure. But after the past 10 years in Gainesville, Florida, I am much more aware of the dangers of skin cancer, sunburn, and heatstroke. If I go out in the sun, I wear a visor; lightweight, no-slip sunglasses designed for running; and a sunscreen with a sun protection factor (SPF) of at least 15. Apply sunscreen to all exposed areas of your skin at least 15 minutes before going out. Try the special sunscreens made for sports. Men are usually not inclined to use creams, but one man I know developed skin cancer after running for years during his lunch break—without his shirt on. Because of the sun's intensity, the experts say that it's best to avoid exercising between the hours of 10:00 A.M. and 2:00 P.M.

Stitches. Stitches are common in any activity that involves running. They are more common among unfit people, but sometimes they can occur if you eat right before running or exercising or suck in too much air without expelling it. According to *Runner's World* magazine, the pain also can come from the force of the abdominal organs tugging at the diaphragm.

While a painful stitch is occurring, focus on forcefully exhaling your breath. If that doesn't help, try bending over to relax the site of the stitch and applying pressure to the spot. If you are prone to stitches, concentrate on breathing from the belly and relaxing your breathing, especially when you're running hard. Finally, strengthen your abdominal muscles. Strong abs can keep your organs more firmly in place so that they don't tug so hard on your diaphragm.

Stomach cramps. The few times I have experienced stomach cramps have been in warm-weather races when I drank more than my stomach could handle. Stomach cramps occur often in sports such as running, where you jump up and down. They also occur when the body cannot absorb fluid, causing it to sit in the stomach. When you are drinking in an endurance activity such as a marathon, remember that "a little a lot is better than a lot a little." By consuming small amounts of fluid over a longer period of time, you'll be less likely to cramp up and your body will absorb the fluid more easily. Also, I found it useful to practice drinking during training to get used to running with fluids.

Diarrhea. Diarrhea during exercise is more common than you might think, but for obvious reasons, no one talks openly about it. After clinics, people often come up to me privately for advice about diarrhea, knowing that I went public with this particular problem.

The 1984 New York City Marathon was a hot one. To combat dehydration during the race, I was drinking a lot—too

Tips from the Top

Pain is a part of life for every athlete or exerciser. It's a consequence of using your body and testing its limits. But how do you know when that pain has gone beyond a mere ache here and there?

With experience, you will intuitively know the difference between pain and injury. Beginners or those adding a new exercise or intensity level almost always experience delayed muscle soreness and overall stiffness, which usually last for one to three days. Pain is different, though. If I feel pain, I pay close attention. If it disappears during exercise after I've warmed up, I keep going but monitor the pain closely. That's because many injuries can begin this way.

An injury tends to be more intense than a pain. It is point specific and does not subside. It is more of a throbbing pain than a diffuse discomfort. If you suspect an injury, do *not* continue your activity. Treat it with rest, ice, compression, and elevation (RICE). If this does not help within three to five days, seek professional medical advice.

much, in fact. In the middle of the race, I had diarrhea. When you are running a major race and are in the lead, you don't stop to go to the bathroom. To me, needing to relieve myself was a detail—I had to get rid of the distraction in order to focus on the race. I did what I had to do while continuing to run, and my problem was visible to everyone. Someone passed me a napkin, and I cleaned myself as well as I could while running. The same thing had happened in the London Marathon in 1983. That time, it was from an upset stomach caused by some anti-inflammatory medicine I had taken. But I went on to win that race in world record time.

You don't have to be in the midst of competition, or even in the nervous state that precedes it, to experience this problem. Diarrhea can happen during regular training as well. Those of us who have had it usually have tried everything to prevent it. What eventually helped me was taking antidiarrhea medication. You also might experiment with when and what you eat. Don't eat right before exercising. Also try eating less fiber or less food before exercising.

Frequent urination, or incontinence. Urinary incontinence, which can be aggravated by exercise, is known to affect some 13 million Americans, most of them women. Some women suffer a weakening of the pelvic muscles after childbirth or with age, but also as a result of activities such as frequent, high-impact aerobics. Try strengthening the pelvic muscles with Kegel's exercises: Simply clench and unclench the muscles you use to control urination. The more you clench them, the more you'll strengthen them. Try this regimen: Do a short clench, then relax; do another clench and try to hold it for 10 to 15 seconds. Do 10 of these exercises three times a day, gradually increasing the number over time. You can do these exercises anytime, anywhere.

Impact injuries. When you're running or even walking, you are vulnerable to the possibility of impact injuries, such as shinsplints and even stress fractures. To help minimize this danger, I've worn orthotics—custom-made shoe inserts constructed by a podiatrist—for years. Because I walk a lot, I also wear a heel cup. You can purchase these shock-absorbing heel inserts, or full insoles, at running or sporting goods stores.

Colds and flu. I was one of those students who was never absent from school. I can't recall when I last had the flu, and my last fever was probably 15 years ago. In fact, in my entire career, I never missed a competition because of illness.

Why have I been so lucky? Part of it must be genetic: My entire family is unusually healthy. In addition, even when I was training hard, I never lived recklessly. I made sure to get enough sleep, eat properly, and stick to my routine. We can't always control illness, though. If you do get sick, it is important *not* to try to train through your illness. Take a day or two off. Some people feel that they can't break their exercise routine. Experts say that if it's a minor illness, you can continue to exercise, but lightly. The great miler Eamonn Coghlan has his own rule: If his symptoms are above the throat—a stuffy nose, sneezing—he exercises lightly. If his symptoms are in or below the throat—especially chest congestion, coughing, a weak feeling in the legs, sweating, or a temperature—he doesn't. If you're sick, exercising can suppress the immune system, making you even more vulnerable to illnesses such as bronchitis and pneumonia. In extreme cases, it can lead to heart damage.

Chronic fatigue syndrome (CFS). This condition, which has been recognized only in the past decade, is a real risk for the busy exerciser. In the past, it was viewed as a psychosomatic illness, but for those who have it, it is far from being all in their heads. CFS is often found in motivated, driven people. Sometimes a virus will spark it, but often heavy stress or pressure can trigger it, too.

One athlete who has had CFS is Peter McColgan, a world-class runner. In 1987, McColgan, who is now 34, got the flu. Instead of backing off, he kept on training. First, the quality of his training suffered. Then his health deteriorated to the point where he was tired, sleepy, and depressed. Worse still, he would breath hard even while jogging. His first solution to the problem was to stop running for nearly two months. But when he started up again, there was no change.

Although he tried everything from herbal treatments to megadoses of vitamins, only time seemed to help. The illness lasted for 18 months. McColgan was lucky. He came back and represented Great Britain in the 3000-meter steeplechase at the World Championships in 1991. But he emphasizes that his recovery was a gradual process. Looking back, he says that he should have gone to the doctor after feeling run-down for two weeks, not two months. Although it's not easy, he says, it's important to try to reduce negative stress and to back off training when necessary. Exercise can be a stress reliever, but if it becomes an additional stress, you should probably reevaluate what you're doing.

About the Authors

The career of Norway's Grete Waitz is legendary. As one of the world's top athletes, her accomplishments include nine wins in the New York City Marathon; 1984 Olympic silver medalist in the marathon; 1983 World Championship gold medalist in the marathon; five wins in both the World Cross-Country Championships and the Women's Mini-Marathon in New York City. She was the first woman to break 2:30 in the marathon, and she set four world records in the event, including the first time she ever ran the distance. Waitz is largely credited as being a major force behind the addition of the women's marathon to the Olympics in 1984. Before beginning her road racing career, Waitz was a 1972 and 1976 Olympian on the track and a two-time world record holder in the 3000 meters.

Eight separate times, Waitz was ranked as the top female runner at various distances from 1500 meters to the marathon. She became the first athlete to receive the St. Olav's Medal for outstanding citizenship when the king of Norway presented it to her in 1982. She also has been awarded the Volvo Prize, given annually to the best sports person in the Nordic countries, and the Monique Berlieux Prize, given by the French Academy of Sports. Waitz was the first non-French person to receive this honor.

In 1991, *Runner's World* magazine's international panel of experts voted Waitz the world's best female distance runner in the past quarter century. There is a bronze statue of Waitz outside the famous Bislett Stadium in her native Oslo. A copy of this statue is located at the Norwegian pavilion at Walt Disney World's Epcot Center in Orlando, Florida.

Since her retirement from competitive running, Waitz has worked on promoting health and fitness worldwide. In 1984, she established the Grete Waitz Run for women in Oslo. This is the largest women's road race in the world, with 45,000 participants. She also has focused on using exercise to promote better health and self-esteem among members of various disadvantaged and charitable groups.

Waitz is co-author of *World Class* (Warner Books, 1984). In 1996, she received an honorary doctorate of humane letters from Iona College in New Rochelle, New York. In April 1997, a Grete Waitz postage stamp, commemorating all sports since World War II, was issued in Norway. Waitz is only the third living Norwegian, along with the king and queen, to have such a stamp.

Grete and her husband, Jack, divide their time between Oslo and Gainesville, Florida.

Gloria Averbuch is a running and fitness writer and the author of six books, including *World Class* with Grete Waitz and the *New York Road Runners Club Complete Book of Running* with Fred Lebow, now in its third printing. She is a features editor for *New York Running News* and has been a consultant for the New York Road Runners Club since 1979. Her regular broadcasts on running and fitness can be heard on WABC radio in New York City.

A lifelong athlete and competitive runner, Averbuch lives in Upper Montclair, New Jersey, with her husband, Paul Friedman, and their two daughters, Yael and Shira.

Photo Credits

Page 4: Courtesy of Grete Waitz
Page 5: Courtesy of Grete Waitz
Page 6: Courtesy of Grete Waitz
Page 7: Harrison Funk
Page 8, top: Gloria Averbuch
Page 8, bottom: Tony Duffy/Allsport
Page 9: Courtesy of Grete Waitz
Page 10: Courtesy of Grete Waitz
Page 11: Courtesy of Grete Waitz
Page 12: Gloria Averbuch
Page 13: Liz Reap/*Runner's World*

Index

Underscored page references indicate boxed text. *Italic* page references indicate photographs. **Boldface** page references indicate main discussion of topic.